D0914744

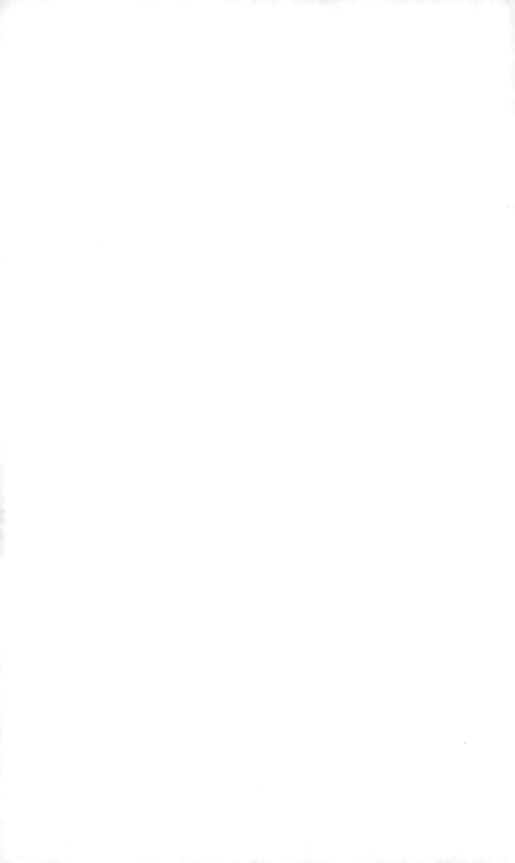

ECONOMIC EVALUATION IN U.S. HEALTH CARE:

PRINCIPLES AND APPLICATIONS

Laura T. Pizzi, PharmD, MPH
Associate Director, Research

Jennifer H. Lofland, PharmD, MPH, PhD
Research Assistant Professor

Department of Health Policy
Jefferson Medical College
Thomas Jefferson University
Philadelphia, Pennsylvania

JONES AND BARTLETT PUBLISHERS
Sudbury, Massachusetts
BOSTON   TORONTO   LONDON   SINGAPORE

World Headquarters
Jones and Bartlett Publishers
40 Tall Pine Drive
Sudbury, MA 01776
978-443-5000
info@jbpub.com
www.jbpub.com

Jones and Bartlett Publishers Canada
6339 Ormindale Way
Mississauga, Ontario L5V 1J2
Canada

Jones and Bartlett Publishers International
Barb House, Barb Mews
London W6 7PA
United Kingdom

Jones and Bartlett's books and products are available through most bookstores and online booksellers. To contact Jones and Bartlett Publishers directly, call 800-832-0034, fax 978-443-8000, or visit our website www.jbpub.com.

Substantial discounts on bulk quantities of Jones and Bartlett's publications are available to corporations, professional associations, and other qualified organizations. For details and specific discount information, contact the special sales department at Jones and Bartlett via the above contact information or send an email to specialsales@jbpub.com.

Production Credits

Executive Editor: Jack Bruggeman
Production Director: Amy Rose
Production Editor: Jenny McIsaac
Marketing Manager: Emily Ekle
Associate Marketing Manager:
  Laura Kavigian

Editorial Assistant: Katilyn Crowley
Cover Design: Kristin E. Ohlin
Cover Image: © Photos.com
Composition: Jason Miranda
Printing and Binding: Malloy
Cover Printing: Malloy

Library of Congress Cataloging-in-Publication Data
Economic evaluation in U.S. health care : principles and applications / [edited by] Laura T. Pizzi and Jennifer H. Lofland.
  p. ; cm.
Includes bibliographical references.
ISBN-13: 978-0-7637-2746-6 (hardcover)
1. Medical care, Cost of—United States—Evaluation. 2. Medical care—United States—Cost effectiveness. 3. Medical economics—United States.
[DNLM: 1. Costs and Cost Analysis—methods—United States. 2. Delivery of Health Care—economics—United States. 3. Evaluation Studies—United States. 4. Quality of Life—United States. W 74 AA1 E19 2006] I. Pizzi, Laura T. II. Lofland, Jennifer H.
RA410.53.E242 2006
362.1'068'1--dc22
                              2005012163

Printed in the United States of America
09 08 07 06 05   10 9 8 7 6 5 4 3 2 1

To Daniel and Jillian, may you lead healthy and productive lives — LP

To Sarah and Joseph, for bringing new purpose and joy to my life — JHL

CONTENTS

Chapter 1   An Overview of the Economic Evaluation
of Healthcare Interventions **1**
Sara Poston, Laura T. Pizzi, and Jennifer H. Lofland

Chapter 2   Measuring Economic Outcomes **15**
Shreekant Parasuraman, Christopher Salvador, and Kevin D. Frick

Chapter 3   Health-Related Quality of Life and Health Utility **41**
Christine Weston and Dong-Churl Suh

Chapter 4   Health-Related Productivity **63**
Nikita Patel, Jennifer H. Lofland, and Laura T. Pizzi

Chapter 5   Adjustments within Economic Evaluation **83**
Craig S. Roberts and Daniel Polsky

Chapter 6   The Industry's Involvement in Economic Evaluation **101**
Dennis Meletiche, Feride Frech, and Laura T. Pizzi

Chapter 7   Formulary Decision-Maker Perspectives:
Responding to Changing Environments **113**
Alan Lyles

Chapter 8 The U.S. Regulator's Perspective in Determining
and Improving the Value of Healthcare Interventions **143**
Richard G. Stefanacci and Jennifer H. Lofland

Chapter 9   The Future of Economic Evaluation within the United States **157**

Jeffrey Clough, Al Crawford, and David B. Nash

FOREWORD

Donald M. Steinwachs, PhD
Director, Professor and Chair
Department of Health Policy and Management
Johns Hopkins Bloomberg School of Public Health
Baltimore, MD

The twentieth century saw life expectancy increase by fifty percent in the United States as advances in public health controlled infectious disease epidemics and advances in medicine provided treatments for infectious and chronic diseases. The twenty-first century will offer comparable opportunities and challenges as the last century did, but for very different reasons. Chronic diseases and health risks associated with modern lifestyles are the new public health threats. While science is providing insights into the causes of chronic diseases and developing innovative treatments at an ever increasing pace, we are being challenged at all levels of the health system to use the products of science well and to achieve the greatest benefits for the public.

Translating the advances in public health and medical sciences into services and programs will mean making choices, whether at the level of the policymakers, providers of healthcare services in the community, or individual consumers and patients. These choices will have consequences both for people's health and for the economies of the United States and other countries. It is reasonable to expect there will be ever increasing opportunities to invest greater proportions of the economic wealth of countries in health services. How big a health benefit is needed to justify greater expenditures? What tools and information are available to make informed decisions about adoption of new health technologies?

This book provides the reader with an understanding of our capacity to use economic evaluation methods to support decision-makers. The tools are designed to be tailored to the decision-maker, measuring costs and benefits appropriate to the decision. The book provides a solid foundation for the public health professional who seeks to understand, interpret, and apply the tools of economic evaluation. For the decision-maker who is the ultimate user of the information, the book provides informative examples of the application of economic evaluation methods from the perspectives of the pharmaceutical industry and health plans making decisions about formularies. Examples drawn from the pharmaceutical industry are particularly timely with the implementation of the Medicare pharmacy benefit in 2006.

Some might question why we need formal methods or tools to provide guidance to decision-makers? Health professionals, whether they are providers, managers, or health policy-analysts, historically have relied on experience, consultation from experts, and limited economic information. Health services research evidence shows consistently that the U.S. healthcare system is failing to provide high quality care. National studies have found chronic disease care meets quality standards about half of the time or less. International comparison of the United States to other industrialized countries has shown the United States to be the highest cost system in the world with comparatively poorer health outcomes. One response to the mounting evidence has been national and international efforts to promote "evidence-based practices" by health care providers. There is a more recent movement to promote "evidence-based management" and increasingly scientific evidence is being used to shape and advocate for health policy. To achieve the goal of a health system that ensures high quality at a reasonable cost, all decision-makers need to have access to relevant scientific evidence.

In the Medicare Modernization Act of 2003, there was clear recognition of the need to invest in improved information for healthcare decision-makers. The Act authorized funding comparative effectiveness studies to provide information that is largely unavailable on the costs and benefits of alternative treatments for specific conditions. This is a critical next step; however, this is not sufficient. Investments will need to be made to educate decision-makers about the use and interpretation of economic evaluation information and to create systems that make the information accessible at the time decisions need to be made. This book fills a critical need in educating the public health professional who provides information to decision-makers and/or creates systems that make decision-relevant information available to users.

PREFACE

David B. Nash, MD, MBA
The Dr. Raymond C. and Doris N.
Grandon Professor of Health Policy
Chairman, Department of Health Policy
Jefferson Medical College
Philadelphia, PA

Healthcare choices are complex. As Americans, we have come to expect that decisions made by our physicians and health plans are based on how effective a test or treatment is in diagnosing or treating disease. However, since increasing healthcare costs are now crippling many U.S. employers and other payers, it is clear that economics will have to play a bigger role in both designing healthcare benefits and in patient care decision making.

With the passage of the Medicare Modernization Act of 2003, which expanded the scope of Medicare to include a prescription drug benefit, it is estimated that federal and state governments will pay for more than half of all health care through the Medicare and Medicaid programs. This marks a major shift as it opens the door for the government to use its purchasing power to require economic evaluation when making coverage decisions.

From my vantage point as Chairman of the Department of Health Policy at Jefferson Medical College, I am keenly aware that all healthcare practitioners and administrators will require a basic understanding of economic evaluation in order to navigate through these changing seas. *Economic Evaluation in U.S. Health Care: Principles and Applications* provides current and future pharmacists, physicians, nurses, public health advocates, and healthcare business leaders with the fundamental concepts of economic evaluation and its application in the United States. In contrast to several other texts on the topic, this book is geared toward those who need a basic understanding of economic evaluation, but may not necessarily be completing economic studies themselves. Doctors Pizzi and Lofland have succeeded in making the content both understandable and relevant for those in all facets of U.S. health care. Using case-based learning, each chapter takes the basic economic evaluation methods and tools and allows readers to apply them to reality-based situations. The book represents a compilation of wisdom and tools from contributors who live in the economic evaluation world every day.

I, along with the book's editors and members of my staff, recognize the importance of thoughtful investments in health care—as will the readers of this book. I am extremely proud of Doctors Pizzi and Lofland and am confident that the reader will benefit from their hard work and dedication to the field.

CONTRIBUTORS

Jeffrey Clough
Medical Student
Jefferson Medical College
Philadelphia PA

Albert Crawford, PhD, MBA, MSIS
Assistant Professor
Department of Health Policy
Jefferson Medical College
Philadelphia PA

Feride H. Frech, RPh, MPH
Director, Outcomes Research
Novartis Pharmaceuticals
East Hanover, NJ

Kevin D. Frick, PhD
Associate Professor
Health Policy and Management
Johns Hopkins University
Bloomberg School of Public Health
Baltimore, MD

Jennifer H. Lofland, PharmD, MPH, PhD
Research Assistant Professor
Department of Health Policy
Jefferson Medical College
Philadelphia, PA

Alan Lyles, ScD, MPH
Associate Professor
Health Systems Management, Government
and Public Administration
School of Public Affairs
University of Baltimore
Baltimore, MD

Dennis M. Meletiche, PharmD
Assistant Director, Regional Outcomes Research
(Northeast Division)
Janssen Pharmaceutica, Inc.
Cambridge, MA

David B. Nash, MD, MBA
The Dr. Raymond C. and Doris N. Grandon
Professor of Health Policy
Chairman, Department of Health Policy
Jefferson Medical College
Philadelphia, PA

Shreekant Parasuraman, PhD
Director, Health Outcomes & Disease
Management
Wyeth Pharmaceuticals
St. David, PA

Nikita Mody Patel, PharmD
Global Health Outcomes Fellow—Infectious
Diseases
GlaxoSmithKline
Collegeville, PA

Laura T. Pizzi, PharmD, MPH
Associate Director, Research
Department of Health Policy
Jefferson Medical College
Philadelphia, PA

Daniel E. Polsky, PhD
Research Associate Professor
General Internal Medicine
University of Pennsylvania
Philadelphia, PA

Sara Poston, PharmD
Outcomes Research Fellow
Ortho-McNeil Janssen Scientific Affairs
Titusville, New Jersey

Craig S. Roberts, PharmD, MPA
Outcomes Research Manager
Pfizer, Inc.
New York, NY

Christopher Salvador, PharmD
Global Health Outcomes Fellow—Oncology
GlaxoSmithKline
Collegeville, PA

**Richard G. Stefanacci, DO, MGH, MBA,
AGSF, CMD**
Founding Executive Director
Health Policy Institute
University of the Sciences in Philadelphia
Philadelphia, PA

Dong-Churl Suh, MBA, PhD
Associate Professor
Rutgers College of Pharmacy
College of Pharmacy
Piscataway, NJ

Christine Weston, MSEd, PhD
Project Director
Department of Health Policy
Jefferson Medical College
Philadelphia, PA

Chapter 1

AN OVERVIEW OF THE ECONOMIC EVALUATION OF HEALTHCARE INTERVENTIONS

Sara Poston, PharmD
Laura T. Pizzi, PharmD, MPH
Jennifer H. Lofland, PharmD, MPH, PhD

Overview

In this chapter we will discuss the current and historical context of economic evaluation of healthcare interventions in the United States. In addition, we will describe the importance of study perspective when conducting economic evaluation, explain the difference between efficacy and effectiveness, describe the circumstances in which an economic analysis is relevant, and provide a brief overview of methods discussed in this book.

Learning Objectives

1. To describe a brief history of the use of economic evaluations in health care
2. To understand the majors factors contributing to the large rise in U.S. healthcare expenditures
3. To understand the importance of perspective in an economic evaluation
4. To introduce the five major methods of economic evaluation and how they differ

Keywords

AMCP Format for Formulary Submissions
Chronic disease
Economic evaluation
Effectiveness
Efficacy
Food and Drug Administration Modernization Act of 1997
Healthcare intervention
Healthcare provider organizations
Healthcare stakeholders
Managed care organizations
Insurers
Oregon Initiative
Outcome measures
Panel on Cost-Effectiveness in Health and Medicine
Patients
Payers
Perspective
Pharmacoeconomics
Purchasers
Value

Introduction

The cost of health care in the United States has gained national attention. Costs have escalated to the point where rationing of medical services is sometimes necessary, such as in the case of expensive medications or diagnostic equipment. Evidence of rising healthcare expenditures is widespread.[1] Hogan and colleagues have estimated private expenditures increased by 6.6 percent per insured person in 1999, as compared with increases of 5.1 percent in 1998 and 3.1 percent in 1997.[2] According to the most recent estimates by the U.S. Centers for Medicare and Medicaid Services (CMS), the rate of growth in national health expenditures is projected to grow by 7.8 percent in 2004, still slightly less than 2003 increase of 7.7 percent.[3] However, during the next 10 years, healthcare spending is expected to outpace economic growth. As a result, the healthcare share of gross domestic product (GDP) is projected to increase from 15.3 percent in 2003 to 18.7 percent in 2014.[3] The Medicare drug benefit legislation (excluded from these projections) passed in 2003 is not anticipated to have a large impact on overall national health spending, but it can be expected to cause sizable shifts in payment sources.[3]

Economic evaluation serves as a tool that helps decision makers, whether in the public or private sectors, determine how healthcare dollars should be spent. In this book, we explain the context and methods of economic evaluation of healthcare interventions in the United States. Economic evaluation assists healthcare decision makers in determining the value of medical interventions, whether those interventions are treatments (medications, devices, behavioral counseling, etc.) or diagnostic tests, where the **value** of a healthcare intervention can be thought of as the ratio between its effectiveness (measured through relevant **outcome measures**) and cost.[4] In economic analyses, common outcome measures are clinical improvements (such as blood pressure unit reductions, infections cured, and survival time), patient quality of life, or preferences for each available intervention. Throughout this text, the term **healthcare intervention** refers to any specific method of diagnosing or treating a disease. For example, healthcare interventions related to diagnosis may consist of diagnostic tests (e.g., laboratory or imaging), whereas those related to treatment may include pharmaceuticals, counseling, educational materials, radiation treatments, and the like.

Through the methods of economic evaluation, the costs of two or more healthcare interventions are weighed in relation to their demonstrated **effectiveness**. Although the term *effectiveness* is often used casually in discussions related to health care, it has a specific meaning with respect to economic evaluation. In this context, effectiveness studies are aimed at evaluating an intervention in a real-world setting, are generally observational, include patients from a variety of demographic backgrounds and clinical histories, and may not include a comparison group (the latter being either a placebo or a treatment alternative).[4] In contrast, **efficacy** studies include a comparison group, and patients may be randomized to one of the study groups.[4] Efficacy studies tend to hold a higher level of scientific rigor than effectiveness studies, and results are not generalizable to a patient population as a whole. Although it is generally preferable to use the results of effectiveness studies in economic evaluation, at times this data does not exist. In such cases, results of efficacy studies may serve as a proxy for effectiveness in economic evaluations, and/or models may be constructed to predict the effectiveness based on efficacy data.

Much of the literature on this topic—as well as applications of economic evaluation in the United States—has been largely focused on pharmaceuticals. As such, sections of this book are specific to the economic evaluation of drug treatments. However, it is important for the reader to bear in mind that the basic methods of economic evaluation can be applied to any type of healthcare intervention.

History of Economic Evaluation in the United States

In the 1970s, the economic evaluation of healthcare services became an academic interest.[5] However, inconsistency in the approaches used to carry out such evaluations led to confusing and often conflicting results. Because of a lack of uniformity in approach, these early economic analyses were of limited use in aiding decisions about which treatments to fund and for whom.

One example of the early and ambitious use of economic evaluation occurred through the **Oregon Initiative** in 1989, when that state, attempting to provide health insurance to all its citizens, relaxed the eligibility requirements for Medicaid coverage.[6, 7] A list of diseases and corresponding treatments was constructed by groups of medical experts and citizens, with treatments then prioritized according to the cost of each in relation to expected effectiveness. The attempt to use economic evaluation as a means of informing coverage decisions was criticized by the public, because some cheaper, nonlifesaving procedures (such as teeth-capping) were prioritized over costly potentially lifesaving treatments (such as appendectomy). The first draft of the priority list was rejected, and a final prioritized list of procedures was created that did not explicitly use costs in determining the ranking. The initiative was a bold and innovative approach that many believe, while technically flawed, was a step in the right direction in terms of incorporating costs into the discussion of healthcare coverage.

In 1993, the U.S. Public Health Service (USPHS) recognized the need for consensus on methods for economic evaluation, specifically cost-effectiveness analysis (CEA). CEA is used to weigh the costs of treatment alternatives with their clinical effectiveness. The USPHS convened a group of 13 nongovernment scientists and scholars with expertise in economic evaluation, collectively referred to as the **Panel on Cost-Effectiveness in Health and Medicine**.[8] The objectives of the panel were to:

1. assess the state of the science in cost-effectiveness analysis,
2. identify methodological inconsistencies and fragilities in the technique,
3. foster consensus, where possible (with respect to standardizing the conduct of studies), and
4. propose steps that can be taken to address remaining issues and uncertainties in the methodology.

The resulting recommendations were compiled in what many refer to as the *Gold Book* or officially, *Cost-Effectiveness in Health and Medicine*.[8]

With the passage of the **Food and Drug Administration Modernization Act of 1997** (FDAMA; discussed further in Chapter 8), the U.S. Food and Drug

Administration (FDA) became involved in regulating the dissemination of economic information by pharmaceutical manufacturers. Specifically, FDAMA allowed manufacturers to disseminate economic information about their products to large purchasers of those products, such as managed care organizations, hospital formulary committees, and the public itself. Under Section 114 of the act, "Healthcare economic information provided to a formulary committee, or other similar entity, in the course of the committee or the entity carrying out its responsibilities for the selection of drugs for managed care or other similar organizations, shall not be considered to be false or misleading . . . if the healthcare economic information directly relates to an indication approved."[9] However, the distribution of economic information to influence the prescribing behavior of individual physicians was prohibited. FDAMA symbolized the increasing importance of providing information to healthcare insurers and administrators about the true value of products.

A more recent milestone in the evolution of economic evaluation in the United States is the publication of guidelines from the Academy of Managed Care Pharmacy (AMCP) in 2000. Known as the **AMCP Format of Formulary Submissions**, these guidelines detail the information that healthcare provider organizations (e.g., hospitals, managed care plans, pharmacy benefit managers) need to evaluate the clinical, economic, and humanistic attributes of a specific drug relative to other treatment alternatives.[10] The AMCP format (discussed further in chapter 7) also provides guidance on the construction of an economic model aimed at informing these providers of the cost of treatment alternatives relative to effectiveness.

The Major Forces Driving U.S. Healthcare Costs

Aging of the U.S. Population

A growing population of elderly Americans poses a significant burden on the U.S. healthcare system. As result of both decreasing fertility rates and increasing life expectancy, the population is growing more slowly, with an increase in the ratio of elderly Americans to those who are of working age. This ratio will most certainly continue to rise as the Baby Boomer generation reaches retirement. By the year 2025, the number of Americans age 65 years and older is estimated to exceed 62 million, compared to 35 million in 2000, with almost 82 million Americans projected to be in this age category by 2050.[11, 12] Coupled with this, the growth rate of the U.S. working age population is expected to shrink by 50 percent by the year 2030.[13]

The Burden of Chronic Disease

Chronic disease has been defined as

> a disease that has one or more of the following characteristics: is permanent;
> leaves residual disability; is caused by nonreversible pathological alteration;
> requires special training of the patient for rehabilitation; or may be expected to
> require a long period of supervision, observation, or care.[14]

During the past century, major public health advances such as improved sanitation and antibiotics led to the containment of many infectious diseases, which contributed to an increased life expectancy of Americans.[15] As a consequence of this longevity and of unhealthy lifestyles,[16] chronic diseases have emerged as the main causes of mortality in the U.S. population (Table 1-1).[17]

Table 1-1 Leading Causes of Death in the United States, 2001

Cause of Death	Deaths in 2001
Heart Diseases	700,142
Cancer	553,768
Cerebrovascular Diseases (such as Stroke)	163,538
Chronic Lower Respiratory Diseases	123,013
Unintentional Injuries	101,537
Diabetes Mellitus	71,372
ALL CAUSES	**2,416,425**

Source: Adapted from Health, United States, 2003.[18] National Center for Health Statistics, United States Centers for Disease Control and Prevention.

New Technologies

Another significant healthcare cost driver is the availability of new technologies to improve the diagnosis or treatment of disease. Not only are strides being made to cure illness, but the invention of many new testing procedures and technologies have enabled physicians to diagnose problems more frequently—and often earlier in the disease process. Innovations such as magnetic resonance imaging (MRI) and positron emission tomography (PET) scanning are examples of such technologies. Although new diagnostic and treatment interventions have significantly advanced the safety and success of healthcare delivery in medical fields, particularly cardiology and oncology, overuse of these technologies when cheaper methods are appropriate is an inefficient use of healthcare resources.[19, 20]

The proliferation of prescription drug products is also straining healthcare budgets and has given rise to an entire subspecialty area of economic evaluation known as **pharmacoeconomics**. Although the rate of growth in pharmaceutical expenditures has slowed during recent years (increased by 13.2 percent in 2002 versus 15 percent in 2000 and 18 percent in 2001), the high price of pharmaceuticals is still a major concern for those involved in public policy and public health. Drugs that represent major innovations in treating disease, also referred to as innovator drugs, contribute the most to pharmaceutical expenditures.[21, 22]

With the exception of health insurance premium payments, prescription drug expenses represent the largest component of out-of-pocket spending on health care.[23] Drug products, especially in the areas of oncology and cardiovascular disease, account for nearly 11 percent of every healthcare dollar spent.[22] On the other hand, the cost of pharmaceuticals may be offset if the drug therapy reduces the patient's need for outpatient medical visits and hospitalizations—or reduces the time they miss from work.

In addition, certain drug therapies may significantly improve a patient's quality of life. A literature review examining drug therapy in asthma, diabetes, heart failure, and migraine showed that prescription drug costs for these conditions were offset by gains in quality of life, as well as decreased use of other medical services.[24] Whether pharmaceutical treatments are actually worth the investment is a major area of concern for public health policy makers. This is where economic analysis of treatment alternatives is necessary in order to quantify each drug's benefits in relation to their cost.

Labor Shortages

Shortages in the number of healthcare workers also drive healthcare costs through wage inflation. Wage inflation has tremendous potential to impact the budgets of healthcare institutions, which in turn must pass the costs on to insurers and patients. Perhaps the most concerning profession is nursing, whose labor shortage permeates both the inpatient and outpatient care sectors. There are nearly 2.7 million nurses in the United States—by far the largest segment of the healthcare workforce.[25] Troubling trends in the profession may lead to increased healthcare spending. Specifically, a 2000 census of the U.S. nursing population found that the average age of a registered nurse was 45.2 years old, with only 9 percent of nurses under the age of 30.[25] It is estimated that more than a million new and replacement nurses will be needed in the United States by the year 2010.[26] A shortage of pharmacists and physicians exists as well.[27, 28] As a result of these shortages, wage rates within these professions have increased in some regions, especially in rural areas.[29]

Consumers' Demand for Choice

Managed care organizations (MCOs) emerged in the United States during the 1990s, as part of an attempt to harness healthcare spending. At that time, MCOs held the promise that investments in preventative care and restrictions of patients' choice in healthcare providers would decrease medical expenses. Although MCOs did reduce healthcare insurance premiums, U.S. consumers were resistant to the rigidity of closed provider networks.[30] Hence, less restrictive forms of health insurance (such as preferred provider organizations and point of service plans) grew in popularity during the late 1990s and early 2000s.[30] Not surprisingly, these more flexible plans have resulted in increased healthcare spending on the part of both healthcare purchasers (primarily employers and the U.S. government) as well as patient consumers, leading to renewed interest in economic evaluation as a tool to curb expenditures.

The Importance of Perspective in Economic Evaluation

The **perspective** of an economic evaluation defines the point of view for assessing costs and outcomes included in the study. Both the costs and outcomes of an economic analysis can be vastly different depending on viewpoint; it is perceived, though from a public health standpoint, that the perspective of the U.S. society as a whole is most relevant. In circumstances where the societal perspective is not possible or relevant to the organization conducting the assessment, economic evaluation is typically tailored to include only the costs and outcomes that are relevant to that organization. **Healthcare stakeholders** are those who have an interest or "stake" in a particular healthcare program or agenda. In the United States, the major healthcare stakeholders interested in economic evaluation are as follows:

1. **Purchasers** that buy healthcare services on behalf of a large population of patients, such as the federal government, state governments, and employers. Also referred to as **payers**.
2. **Insurers**, particularly MCOs and pharmacy benefit managers (PBMs), that administer medical and/or pharmaceutical benefits to patients.
3. **Healthcare provider organizations** that provide medical services directly to patients, such as hospitals, healthcare systems, clinics, and group medical practices.
4. **Patients** who receive care from healthcare providers.

Each of these stakeholders possesses a specific perspective that determines both the method and content of an economic evaluation.

When Is Economic Evaluation Warranted?

Although the increased cost of a diagnostic or treatment intervention may stimulate interest in conducting an economic evaluation to compare its costs and effects to other treatment alternatives, it is important to note that economic evaluation is not always warranted. Consider an example where there are two different treatment interventions of interest (Figure 1-1). If one intervention has a greater effectiveness and lower cost than the other, an evaluation is not necessary because the cheaper and more effective treatment is an obvious choice. When interventions have both an equal effectiveness and an equal cost, economic evaluation may be of interest, but will be of limited value in making decisions as to which should be offered. However, when the intervention is either more effective but has a higher cost or is less effective but has a lower cost than its comparator, an economic evaluation is essential in order to quantify the difference between costs and outcomes between the two alternatives. Because new interventions typically cost more than existing options, the former scenario is frequently the case.

Figure 1-1 Decision Matrix for Determining If an Economic Evaluation Comparing Two Medical Interventions Is Warranted

		Effect		
		High	**Equal**	**Low**
Cost	**High**	Yes	No	No
	Equal	No	Neutral	No
	Low	No	No	Yes

Source: Adapted from Reeder CE. Overview of pharmacoeconomics and pharmaceutical outcomes evaluations. *Am J Health Syst Pharm.* 1995;52(19 Suppl 4):S5–8.[31]

■ A Brief Overview of Methods and Organization of This Book

There are five major methods of economic evaluation (Table 1-2), that are discussed in Chapters 2 and 3 of this book. Although the methods vary and the outcome of interest may be measured in different ways (i.e., dollars, dollars per year of life saved, etc.), the aim of all methods is to determine the costs attributable to medical conditions and/or which health intervention is the most valuable among those that are being compared. Cost of illness and burden of illness analyses are excluded from this table because these types of studies generally present costs of a disease or condition, without consideration of outcome.

Table 1-2 Methods of Economic Evaluation

Method	Costs Units	Benefit Units	Location in This Book
Cost-Consequence Analysis (CCA)	Monetary	Broad range of outcomes presented in natural units	Chapter 2
Cost-Minimization Analysis (CMA)	Monetary	None, because effectiveness is assumed to be equal for both interventions	Chapter 2
Cost-Effectiveness Analysis (CEA)	Monetary	Clinical outcomes, such as blood pressure units or infections cured	Chapter 2
Cost-Utility Analysis (CUA)	Monetary	Utility to patients, such as quality adjusted life years (QALYs)	Chapters 2 and 3
Cost-Benefit Analysis (CBA)	Monetary	Monetary (the value of the effectiveness measure is converted to dollars)	Chapter 2

Source: Adapted from *Principles of Pharmacoeconomics*, Third Edition, edited by Bootman et al., p. 6 with permission from Harvey Books Company.

Chapters 4 and 5 pertain to concepts related to economic evaluation. Specifically, Chapter 4 explains how health-related work productivity (work lost due to a disease or health condition) is measured; Chapter 5 explains why costs and outcomes must be adjusted for time, as well as when and why risk adjustment is important when conducting an economic evaluation. Latter chapters of the book (Chapters 7 and 8) summarize the perspectives and application of economic evaluation by different U.S. healthcare stakeholders, with the final chapter (Chapter 9) discussing future directions in this field.

In today's healthcare environment, economic evaluation gives various stakeholders the tools to determine the best value for healthcare dollars. These tools are especially useful to those in public health, pharmacy, and medical professions who are responsible for making treatment decisions.

Case Study

The following case study provides an example of the relevance of economic evaluation in comparing the costs and effects of treatments for colon cancer. This case was adapted from Schrag, *New England Journal of Medicine, 2004.*[32]

Chemotherapy for metastatic colon cancer serves as an example of the high cost of new medical technology. Decades ago, the outlook for patients diagnosed with this condition was bleak, with a survival time after diagnosis of 8 months.

When fluorouracil, a chemotherapeutic agent, was introduced in the 1960s, average survival increased to 12 months. Other chemotherapeutic agents introduced in the 1990s have further increased survival to 21 months, and two new agents, both biotechnology products recently available, are anticipated to increase survival beyond 21 months.

However, the costs of newer treatment regimens are extremely high. An 8-week course of first-line chemotherapy combined with either of the two new biotechnology products ranges from over $21,000 to over $30,000. Before these biotechnology breakthroughs, the cost of an 8-week, first-line chemotherapy regimen ranged from $10,000 to $12,000. Most patients will continue therapy up to several months, making these numbers an underestimate of the true cost. In addition to direct drug costs, the cost for drugs to manage the toxic side effects of chemotherapy must be considered, along with costs for nursing administration, time and the cost of having a pharmacist prepare the drugs for administration. If the patient has to be admitted to the hospital ward to receive chemotherapy, the costs will be significantly higher.

Economic evaluation could be used as a method in determining the value of such high-cost interventions. Insurance companies could use a cost-benefit or cost-effectiveness analysis to determine whether or not to cover such treatments. A cost-utility analysis, which uses quality-of-life measurements in the value equation, would be useful in deciding which interventions will be valuable to patients, purchaser, and society as a whole.

Study/Discussion Questions

1. What major factors have contributed to rising U.S. healthcare expenditures?
2. What is perspective and how is it important to economic evaluation?
3. Under what circumstances is an economic evaluation of diagnostic or treatment alternatives for a given disease or condition warranted?
4. What are the five major methods of economic evaluation and how do they differ?

Suggested Readings/Web Sites

Academy of Managed Care Pharmacy. Format for Formulary Submissions, Version 2.0. Available at: www.amcp.org/data/nav_content/formatv20%2E.pdf.

Food and Drug Modernization Act of 1997 (FDAMA), Section 114. Available at: www.fda.gov/cder/guidance/105-115.htm.

Gold M, Siegel J, Russel L, Weinstein M. *Cost-Effectiveness in Health and Medicine.* New York: Oxford Press; 1996.

▌ References

1. Blumenthal D. Controlling healthcare expenditures. *N Engl J Med.* 2001;344(10):766–769.

2. Hogan C, Ginsburg PB, Gabel JR. Tracking healthcare costs: inflation returns. *Health Aff (Millwood).* 2000;19(6):217–223. Available at: http://content.healthaffairs.org/cgi/content/full/hlthaff.w4.79v1/DC1. Accessed December 20, 2004.

3. Heffler S, Smith S, Keehan S, Borger C, Clemens MK, Truffer C. Trends: U.S. health spending projections for 2004–2014. *Health Aff (Millwood).* 2005;w5:74–85. Available at: http://content.healthaffairs.org/cgi/reprint/hlthaff.w5.74v1. Accessed May 10, 2005.

4. Toscani MR, Pizzi LT. Measuring and improving the intervention. In: Patterson R (ed). *Changing Patient Behavior: Improving Outcomes in Health and Disease Management.* San Francisco: Jossey Bass; 2001.

5. Blumenschein K, Johannesson M. Economic evaluation in healthcare. A brief history and future directions. *Pharmacoeconomics.* 1996;10(2):114–122.

6. Ham C. Retracing the Oregon trail: The experience of rationing and the Oregon health plan. *BMJ.* 1998;316(7149):1965–1969.

7. Stason WB. Oregon's bold Medicaid initiative. *JAMA.* 1991;265(17):2237–2238.

8. Gold M, Siegel J, Russel L, Weinstein M. *Cost Effectiveness in Health and Medicine.* New York: Oxford Press; 1996.

9. U.S. Food and Drug Administration. Food and Drug Modernization Act of 1997 (FDAMA), Section 114. Public Law 105-45. Available at: http://www.fda.gov/cder/guidance/105-115.htm. Accessed January 17, 2005.

10. Academy of Managed Care Pharmacy. Format for Formulary Submissions Version 2.0. Available at: http://www.amcp.org/data/nav_content/formatv20%2Epdf. Accessed January 5, 2005.

11. Hetzel L, Smith A. The 65 years and over population: 2000. 2001; U.S. Census Bureau (Publication No. C2KBR/01-10). Available at: http://www.census.gov/prod/2001pubs/c2kbr01-10.pdf. Accessed January 17, 2005.

12. U.S. Census Bureau. Projections of the total resident population by 5-year age groups and sex with special age categories: Middle series, 2025 to 2045. (Report No. NP-T3-F). 2000. Available at: http://www.census.gov/population/projections/nation/summary/np-t3-f.pdf. Accessed January 17, 2005.

13. Greenspan A. Testimony before the special committee on aging, United States Senate. 2003. Available at: http://www.federalreserve.gov/boarddocs/testimony/2003/20030227/default.htm. Accessed January 17, 2005.

14. Academy Health. Glossary of Terms Commonly Used in Healthcare. Washington, DC: Academy Health, 2004. Available at: http://www.academyhealth.org/publications/glossary.pdf. Accessed January 17, 2005.

15. Arias E. United States life tables, 2002. National vital statistics reports: vol 53, no. 6. November 10, 2004. Hyattsville, MD: National Center for Health Statistics (DHHS Publication No. 2005-1120). Avaliable at: http://www.cdc.gov/NCHS/data/nvsr/ nvsr53/nvsr53_06.pdf. Accessed January 17, 2005.

16. World Health Organization. Facts related to chronic diseases. Available at: http://www.who.int/dietphysicalactivity/publications/facts/chronic/en/ Accessed January 17, 2005.

17. U.S. Department of Health and Human Services. Healthy People 2010: Understanding and improving health, 2nd ed. Washington, DC: U.S. Government Printing Office, November 2000. Available at: http://www.phppo.cdc.gov/owpp/docs/library/2000/ HP%202010%20Understanding%20and%20Improving%20Health.pdf. Accessed January 17, 2005.

18. U.S. Department of Health and Human Services. Health, United States, 2003. Washington, DC: U.S. Government Printing Office. (DHHS Publication No. 2003-1232). Available at: http://www.cdc.gov/nchs/data/hus/tables/2003/03hus031.pdf. Accessed January 17, 2005.

19. Alavi A, Kung JW, Zhuang H. Implications of PET based molecular imaging on the current and future practice of medicine. *Semin Nucl Med*. 2004;34(1):56–69.

20. Goldbach-Mansky R, Woodburn J, Yao L, Lipsky PE. Magnetic resonance imaging in the evaluation of bone damage in rheumatoid arthritis: A more precise image or just a more expensive one. *Arthritis Rheum*. 2003;48(3):585–589.

21. Hoffman JM, Shah ND, Vermeulen LC, Hunkler RJ, Hontz KM. Projecting future drug expenditures—2004. *Am J Health Syst Pharm*. 2004;61(2):145–158.

22. Cohen FJ. Macro trends in pharmaceutical innovation. *Nat Rev Drug Discov*. 2005;4:78–84.

23. Centers for Medicare and Medicaid Services. Healthcare Financing Review: Medicare and Medicaid Statistical Supplement, 2001. November 1, 2002. Available at: http://www.cms.hhs.gov/review/supp/. Accessed January 17, 2005.

24. Goldfarb N, Weston C, Hartmann CW, et al. Impact of appropriate pharmaceutical therapy for chronic conditions on direct medical costs and workplace productivity: A review of the literature. *Dis Manag*. 2004;7(1):61–75.

25. Sprately E, Johnson A, Sochalski J, Fritz M, Spencer W. U.S. Department of Health and Human Services. The registered nurse population: Findings from the national sample of registered nurses. 2002. Available at: http://bhpr.hrsa.gov/ healthworkforce/reports/rnsurvey/rnss1.htm. Accessed January 17, 2005.

26. Hecker D. Occupational employment projections to 2010. Monthly Labor Review 2001. Available at: http://www.bls.gov/opub/mlr/2001/11/art4full.pdf/. Accessed January 17, 2005.

27. Cooper RA, Getzen TE, McKee HJ, Laud P. Economic and demographic trends signal an impending physician shortage. *Health Aff (Millwood)*. 2002;21(1):140–154.

28. Report to Congress. The Pharmacist Workforce: A Study of the Supply and Demand for Pharmacists. Health Resources and Services Administration, December 2000. Available at: ftp://ftp.hrsa.gov/bhpr/nationalcenter/pharmacy/pharmstudy.pdf. Accessed January 17, 2005.

29. National Rural Health Association. Policy brief: Healthcare workforce distribution and shortage issues in rural America. 2003. Available at: http://www.nrharural.org/dc/policybriefs/WorkforceBrief.pdf. Accessed January 17, 2005.

30. Kaiser Family Foundation. Employer Health Benefits 2004 Annual Survey. Available at: http://www.kff.org/insurance/7148/loader.cfm?url=/commonspot/security/getfile.cfm&PageID=46206. Accessed January 17, 2005.

31. Reeder CE. Overview of pharmacoeconomics and pharmaceutical outcomes evaluations. *Am J Health Syst Pharm*. 1995;52(19 Suppl 4):S5–8.

32. Schrag D. The price tag on progress: Chemotherapy for colorectal cancer. *N Engl J Med*. 2004;351(4):317–319.

Chapter 2

MEASURING ECONOMIC OUTCOMES

Shreekant Parasuraman, PhD
Christopher Salvador, PharmD
Kevin D. Frick, PhD

Overview

This chapter presents established techniques for measuring economic outcomes, beginning with the introduction of different types and forms of cost followed by the methods of comparing the costs and effects of healthcare interventions. This chapter also includes an introduction to economic modeling and lists criteria that are useful when critiquing economic assessments.

There are generally three types of costs used in economic analyses: direct medical cost, direct nonmedical cost, and indirect costs. Direct medical costs represent the value of medical resources consumed as a direct result of the procedure or event. A direct nonmedical cost is defined as the value of nonmedical goods, services, and other resources spent as a direct result of the event or intervention. Indirect costs usually refer to time lost due to the event (i.e., reduced work productivity, which may also result in a monetary loss for either the individual or their employer). There are also intangible costs that are more difficult to measure, although the contingent market valuation literature attempts to do this.

Different methods of economic evaluation include cost-minimization analysis, cost-consequence analysis, cost-effectiveness analysis, cost-utility analysis, and cost-benefit analysis. In cost-minimization analysis, two or more interventions that have been assumed or shown to have the same effectiveness or to both meet some desired threshold are compared for cost and the least expensive one is recommended for policy consideration. This is the simplest type of economic analysis. Cost-consequence analysis (CCA) is another type of economic assessment in which the costs and outcomes are described and presented as independent components in an itemized table, but no summary measure of effect is used. A cost-effectiveness analysis (CEA) uses a single outcome (even if there are multiple outcomes that might be considered) and the end result is a ratio of the change in cost over the change in effectiveness. Differences between two or more interventions are usually presented using an incremental cost-effectiveness ratio (ICER). Cost-utility analysis (CUA) is a type of cost-effectiveness analyses in which the measure of effectiveness is quality adjusted life years (QALYs). Cost-benefit analysis (CBA) is a form of economic evaluation in which both the incremental cost and benefits of the intervention are measured in monetary units.

The data to calculate the costs related to the interventions under study and the effect of the interventions sometimes come from a randomized trial and other times from models. Models are often an integral part of economic analyses and are useful in the absence of empiric data on the costs and/or effectiveness pertaining to the interventions of interest. The two primary types of models that are used include budget impact models and decision analytic models. Budget impact models are used to predict the budgetary impact of an intervention or treatment. Decision analysis is defined as an explicit, quantitative, systematic approach in which probabilities of each event along with its consequences are stated explicitly. Other, more complex methods of modeling include Markov models and Monte Carlo simulations—both of which can be used to enhance the other types of modeling exercises.

With increasing interest in economic evaluation, tools like the Quality of Health Economic Studies (QHES) instrument have been proposed to assess the quality of economic studies. Although the role, current methods, and reporting of economic assessments are still evolving, measuring economic outcomes will play an increasingly important role in the decision-making process in healthcare.

▮ Learning Objectives

1. To identify and understand different types and forms of cost
2. To describe the five major techniques for conducting economic evaluation
3. To be able to evaluate the quality of economic evaluations

Keywords

Adjusting for inflation
Base case
Budget impact model
Burden of illness
Cost of illness
Chance node
Charges
Cost-benefit analysis
Cost-consequence analysis
Cost-effectiveness analysis
Cost-effectiveness plane
Cost-minimization analysis
Cost-utility analysis
Decision analysis
Decision node
Decision trees
Direct medical costs
Direct nonmedical costs
Discount rate
Discounting
Dominance
Expected value
Incremental cost-effectiveness ratio
Indirect costs
Intangible cost
Ishikawa diagram
Markov models
Modeling
Monte Carlo simulation
Net benefit
Opportunity cost
Payoff
Present value
Reference case
Sensitivity analysis
Terminal node
Utility

▮ Introduction

In order to understand economic analyses, a basic understanding of cost must first be established. There are three types of costs: direct costs, indirect costs, and intangible costs.

Direct medical costs are defined as the total value of healthcare resources consumed (e.g., laboratory tests, medicines, supplies, healthcare personnel, and medical equipment and overheads) while administering the intervention, addressing the side effects, or other current and future consequences linked to it.[1] It includes all types of resources consumed in the delivery of health care, including medical resource utilization and labor. In some cases, where the intervention has long-term effects, direct costs affect both current and future resource use and hence the costs should be considered a "stream" of resource use that can span a defined duration of time. In identifying medical costs, it is also important to distinguish between cost and charges. **Charges** are usually the amount that is billed by the institution (i.e., patient bills).[2] While cost is a direct reflection of the resource expensed, charges are artificial figures that can vary substantially from the true costs.

Direct costs are typically subdivided into direct medical and direct nonmedical costs. **Direct nonmedical costs** are attributed to nonmedical goods, services, and other resources, such as child care or transportation to the healthcare facility. These costs are real but often incidental to receiving care.

Indirect costs consists of three categories of time costs:
1. costs related to the treatment in question that involve the time of patients and unpaid caregivers (such as family members or others not considered to be formal healthcare providers),
2. costs associated with lost or reduced ability to work or to enjoy leisure activities due to morbidity, and
3. lost economic productivity due to death.

All three of these are focused on economic productivity measurement. The unpaid caregivers in the first case can be family or friends providing home care, which can range from a day of help while a stay-at-home parent is suffering from a migraine headache to providing nursing care for a disabled individual or sick child.

An **intangible cost** reflects the value of a patient's pain and suffering due to the disease, drug, or healthcare intervention. Because it is difficult to translate intangible costs into monetary units, measures of pain and suffering are commonly captured using quality-of-life (QOL) instruments or assessing the patient's utility or preference for his or her treatment options. However, there is literature on contingent market valuation that sometimes attempts to assess the value of intangible consequences of illness and medical care.

A useful tool in capturing and organizing cost factors is an Ishikawa diagram. An **Ishikawa diagram**, otherwise known as a cause-and-effect diagram, graphically depicts the relationship between a particular outcome and all of the identified factors contributing to that outcome.[3] In terms of costing, Ishikawa diagrams can organize all cost factors contributing to the total cost of a particular outcome. For example, in a study by Goldfarb and associates, an Ishikawa diagram (Figure 2-1) was used to reflect all cost factors in the diagnosis of Crohn's disease.[4] In this study, all cost factors in the diagnosis of Crohn's were organized into six categories (five direct + one indirect): endoscopy, radiology, laboratory, administration, complications, and indirect costs.

Because of general human impatience and the ability to earn returns on money that has been invested, costs that occur over time are usually expressed in terms of their present value, which differs from the simple sum of the stream of costs because of an adjustment that often involves an interest rate. **Discounting**

Figure 2-1 Ishikawa Diagram of the Cost for the Diagnosis of Crohn's Disease

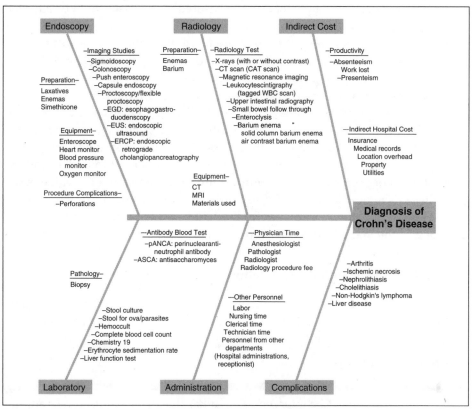

Source: Disease Management Winter 2004. Reprinted with permission from *Disease Management*, published by Mary Ann Liebert, Inc. New Rochelle, NY.

(discussed further in Chapter 5) is a method of adjusting costs and cost savings that occur in the future to their present value. The process of discounting allows expression of the amount of money needed now for a sequence of expenditures over time or the amount a stream of savings over time is worth today. The constant (or rate) used to adjust future costs to reflect present-day values is called the **discount rate** and is often an approximation of a market-based interest rate. The discount rate recommended for use in economic evaluations in the United States is 3 percent.[5] **Present value (P)** is calculated by the following equation where (r) represents the discount rate, (n) represents time in years with this year being represented by $n = 0$, and (F_n) represents the future cost at year n:

$$P = \frac{F_n}{(1 + r)^n}$$

Discounting is generally not required for economic evaluations concerned with a time period of 1 year or less.

It is also important to note that costs measured in the past should be adjusted to the amount of dollars the same use of resources would require today. It is imperative to compare cost values that are consistent with respect to time (i.e., comparing 2004 USD to 2004 USD). This is called **adjusting for inflation**. Adjusting for inflation accounts for expenditures in the past that need to be expressed in today's dollars. This is in contrast to discounting, which summarizes a series of expenditures over time in terms of how much money would be required to have in the bank today. The rates of inflation for healthcare services in the United States can be obtained from the Bureau of Labor Statistics (www.bls.gov).

When conducting an economic evaluation, it is important to understand the concept of an opportunity cost. An **opportunity cost** represents the value of the forfeiting of the next best use of a resource; in other words, the value forgone when choosing not to use resources for the next best alternative. In many cases—but not all—the market price is a good measure of the societal opportunity cost.[1]

Methods of Economic Evaluation

As introduced in Chapter 1, there are five major methods of economic evaluation: cost-minimization analysis, cost-consequence analysis, cost-effectiveness analysis, cost-utility analysis, and cost-benefit analysis.

Cost-Minimization Analysis

In a **cost-minimization analysis** (CMA), the effectiveness of both interventions is considered to be equal. The intervention that has the lower acquisition or administration costs is considered to be the preferred choice. An advantage of using

CMA is its straightforward approach in which the lower cost option would be the best choice. However, two medical interventions are rarely equivalent in real-world settings, and analyses rarely begin as CMAs. Depending on what is meant by equal effectiveness, interventions may not be identical but can differ in various aspects, including end points, side-effect profiles, and QOL.

An example of CMA can be found in a study by Chen and associates that used a CMA of diuretic-based antihypertensive therapy to assess which of several options had the lowest cost of treatment to prevent one adverse outcome related to cardiovascular disease (CVD).[6] While different interventions have a different number needed to treat (NNT) to prevent one adverse outcome, this can be used as the measure of equal effectiveness. The cost, in this case, varied based on a combination of the cost per patient treated and the NNT to prevent an adverse event. The cost to treat enough cases to prevent one adverse event is a function both of the NNT to prevent one adverse event and the cost per treatment. Chen and associates found that the therapy from the Systolic Hypertension in the Elderly Program (SHEP) was associated with the lowest cost of treating the NNT to avoid one adverse outcome.[6]

Cost-Consequence Analysis

Another type of economic assessment is **cost-consequence analysis** (CCA). In CCA, the costs and outcomes are presented as separate components. Generally, CCA presents all types of cost (direct and indirect) and outcomes (QALY, QOL, clinical outcomes). An advantage of CCA is the flexibility for decision makers to choose the cost and outcome of interest in order to tailor the economic assessment to their appropriate situation. Decision makers who value cost-effectiveness analyses but would like more appropriate data may also find this approach useful because they can choose the information of most interest to perform their own cost-effectiveness analysis to closely reflect their concerns. Therefore, one advantage in using CCA is that it can be tailored to all perspectives (such as healthcare payor, patient, provider). Conversely, a perceived disadvantage is leaving the final step in the economic assessment to the decision maker. The relative valuation of different costs and benefits is left to be assigned implicitly by the decision maker rather than being assigned explicitly. To make a decision based on multiple consequences, a weighting system must be devised to determine the importance of the different costs and outcomes with respect to different perspectives. An example of an itemized table used in CCA can be found in Table 2-1.

Cost-Effectiveness Analysis

One of the more widely used economic assessments in the field is **cost-effectiveness analysis** (CEA), which uses natural or physical units as the outcome measure. CEA is used to help understand the relationship between the cost of an intervention and a particular endpoint. The **incremental cost-effectiveness ratio** (ICER) is applied when evaluating a treatment or intervention. ICERs are calculated by dividing the incremental (or extra) cost of the intervention by the incremental (or extra) effectiveness:

$$\text{Incremental Cost-Effectiveness Ratio} = \frac{\text{Extra Cost}}{\text{Extra Effectiveness}}$$

If there is only one intervention, then the "extra" cost and effect is relative to the status quo. Rarely does the status quo have literally zero effect and zero cost. In some cases, there is a new alternative that is less expensive than the status quo;

Table 2-1 Example of a Cost-Consequence Table

	Intervention A		Intervention B	
	Units	Costs	Units	Costs
Direct Medical Costs				
Intervention A/B				
Other medication/Interventions				
Physician office visits				
ER visits				
Hospitalizations				
Home care				
Direct Nonmedical Costs				
Transportation				
Paid caregiver time				
Indirect Nonmedical Costs				
Transportation				
Paid caregiver time				
Indirect Nonmedical Costs				
Patient time missed from work				
Unpaid caregiver time off from work				
Symptom Impact				
Patient distress days				
Patient disability days				
Adverse Events				
Serious adverse events				
Moderate adverse events				
Mild adverse events				
Health-Related Quality-of-Life Impact				
Quality-adjusted life years				
Quality-of-life profile				

Source: Mauskopf JA, Paul JE, Grant DM, Stregachis A. The role of cost consequence analysis in health care decision making. *Pharmacoeconomics.* 1998;13(3):277–288. Reprinted with permission from Adis International.

in that case, the status quo can be compared with the newer, less expensive alternative to determine whether the status quo is effective in light of new choices.

As a more concrete example, when comparing a more expensive intervention (which we will call Intervention B) with a less expensive intervention (which we will call Intervention A), the ICER is calculated as follows:

$$ICER = \frac{(Cost_B - Cost_A)}{(Effect_B - Effect_A)}$$

ICERs will show the change in cost per change in effect. The measure of effectiveness greatly depends on the objectives of the treatments or procedures being evaluated. Effectiveness measures can be absolute clinical end points in a particular study or surrogate end points. Examples of effectiveness measures include blood pressure readings in patients with hypertension, hemoglobin A1C in diabetics, or tumor response rates in patients with cancer. If surrogate outcomes are measured, these are useful only if there is an established relationship with a final outcome.

One of the advantages of CEA is that it quantifies the trade-off between costs and health effects. Furthermore, it measures effectiveness in natural units that are easy for clinicians to understand and interpret. Therefore, physicians can compare two treatments/interventions based on cost and specified outcome end points. Of course, this is also a disadvantage; a cost-effectiveness result can be used only to compare two interventions with the same end point.

One of the disadvantages of CEA is that the results can reflect only one outcome. The primary measure of effect may miss important benefits. Therefore, decision makers are left to decide implicitly how the effects that do not appear in the ratio compare with the effects that do. As with all economic evaluations, restricted perspectives may also be a limitation. For example, a payer perspective that does not include the entire healthcare system can lead to conclusions about which alternatives are economically favorable that would result in cost shifting (i.e., shifting costs to another party). As with other economic assessments, cost data should be consistent across all comparisons with respect to time (discounting) and perspective (societal, payer, patient, etc.)

When there are more than two treatments, ICERs are calculated comparing alternatives two at a time, starting with the least costly intervention. However, not all alternatives necessarily receive consideration after the economic analysis is complete. Alternatives that are dominated are removed from consideration. Strong **dominance** refers to a situation in which one intervention is more effective and less costly than another—the one that is more expensive and less effective is referred to as being dominated. Weak dominance is a situation where the ICER for one option is greater than that of the next, more effective option. In other words, although the next option is more effective and more costly, the next alternative after that is more cost-effective and therefore should be chosen instead of the previous option. Strong dominance involves a simple comparison between two treatments, whereas extended dominance occurs with three or more treatment alternatives. A combination of two alternatives is required to weakly dominate a third. Alternatives that are considered to be dominated should be removed from the decision-making process since they are not considered cost-effective options.

In addition to computing individual ICERs, a **cost-effectiveness plane** (Figure 2-2) may be a useful tool in illustrating the cost-effectiveness of competing interventions and may serve as a double check on the elimination of weakly dominated alternatives. The horizontal axis (x) represents the difference in effect, while the vertical axis (y) represents the difference in cost. There are four quadrants (I–IV) representing different areas of the cost-effectiveness plane. The origin (o) represents the status quo or the treatment standard to which the alternatives are being compared. An alternative (A) intervention can lie anywhere in quadrants I–IV, depending on the difference in cost and effectiveness with respect to the origin (status quo). For example, if the alternative intervention is more costly and more effective, then the coordinates will fall in quadrant I. A line can then be drawn connecting the alternative intervention to the origin. The slope of the line (m) repre-

Figure 2-2 Cost-Effectiveness Plane

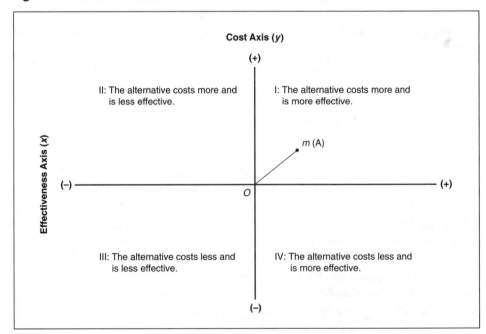

Source: Adapted from Drummond et al: *Methods for the Economic Evaluation of Health Care Programmes*, Second Edition. William C. Black, Medical Decision Making (Vol. 10/No. 3) pp. 212–214, copyright 1990 by Sage Publications. Reprinted by permission of Sage Publications.

sents the cost-effectiveness ratio (change in cost over the change in effectiveness). Alternative interventions that lie in quadrant II are considered dominated by the status quo, while alternative interventions found in quadrant IV is considered to be the opposite (status quo is dominated by the alternative). Drawn this way, if there are more than two alternatives, the line connecting undominated alternatives should become steeper when moving to the right away from the origin.

As discussed in Chapter 1, in 1993 the U.S. Public Health Service convened a panel on cost-effectiveness in health and medicine comprised of 13 nongovernment scientists and scholars with expertise in cost-effectiveness analysis. Their assessment of the current state of knowledge and recommendations has been compiled, which serves as an excellent resource for further reading. Although CEA can be tailored to different perspectives, the panel advised that **reference case** CEAs be based on a societal perspective. The reference case represents an analysis done following all the recommended standards or as many as it is feasible to follow.[5] A summary of major recommendations is provided in Figure 2-3. This is a high, but important standard, for the evaluation of CEAs in the literature.

Figure 2-3 Major Recommendations from the Panel on Cost-Effectiveness in Medicine

---

1. Cost-effectiveness analysis (CEA) is a methodology for evaluating the outcomes and costs of interventions designed to improve health.

2. CEA evaluates a given health intervention through use of a cost-effectiveness ratio.

3. CEA is an aide to decision making, not a complete procedure for making resource allocation decisions in health and medicine, because it cannot incorporate all the values relevant to such decisions.

4. CEA and cost-benefit analysis are complementary, rather than mutually exclusive, forms of analysis. The use of one does not preclude the use of any of the others in a given study.

5. When a CEA is intended to contribute to decisions on the broad allocation of health resources, a reference case analysis should be done to enhance comparability across studies.

6. The reference case is based on the societal perspective. This perspective requires that an analysis consider all health effects and all changes in resource use.

7. The reference case analysis should compare the health intervention of interest to existing practice (the "status quo").

8. The estimates of resource consumption and effects of relevance for a CEA are those for the population or group that is actually affected by the health intervention.

Source: Gold et al., 1996.[5]

An example of a CEA can be found in a study by Khandker and associates that assessed the guidelines for the population at average risk for developing colorectal cancer using a CEA.[8] Because empiric data from clinical trials were not available for all the possible outcomes a subject can experience while having colorectal cancer, a decision analysis model was used.

Khandker and associates used life years saved as the effectiveness outcome and reported results in terms of costs and life-year saved.[8] Table 2-2 adapts their results, lining up alternatives by cost, not including ICERs for dominated alternatives, and focusing only on their "base case" model for the purposes of illustration. Rounding the results to two decimal places, the 3-year flexible sigmoidoscopy result is strongly dominated (it costs more and has a lower measure of effectiveness than annual fecal occult bloodtest) and the four most expensive alternatives are all dominated by the 5-year, double-contrast barium enema. All three nondominated alternatives (other than no screening) appear to be fairly cost-effective when considering the incremental cost-effectiveness of the options. Although there is no absolutely agreed-upon ICER, a cost of less than $100,000 per life year gained is often considered cost-effective. More will be said about this in the section on cost-utility analysis.

Table 2-2 Cost-Effectiveness Estimates for Base Case and Fixed-Length Models, 1994 U.S. Dollars

	Base Case Model		
	Cost ($ Per Person)	Effectiveness	Incremental Cost: Effectiveness Ratio ($)
Baseline (no screening)	643	18.14	—
5-year flexible sigmoidoscopy	1,713	18.23	$11,889
Annual FOBT	2,058	18.24	$34,500
3-year flexible sigmoidoscopy	2,079	18.23	—
5-year double-contrast barium enema	2,577	18.25	$51,900
10-year colonoscopy	2,602	18.25	—
Annual FOBT/5-year flexible sigmoidoscopy	2,639	18.25	—
Annual FOBT/3-year flexible sigmoidoscopy	2,854	18.25	—
5-year colonoscopy	3,906	18.25	—

Source: Adapted from Khandker et al, "A Decision Model and Cost-Effectiveness Analysis of Colorectal Cancer Screening and Surveillance Guidelines for Average-Risk Adults." International Journal of Technology Assessment in Health Care, Vol. 16, Issue 3 (July 2000): 799–810. Reprinted with Permission of Cambridge University Press.

Cost-Utility Analysis

Cost-utility analysis (CUA) is a special application of a cost-effectiveness analysis. In a CUA, the effectiveness is measured in terms of patient preference or the perceived **utility** of the intervention. The perception can be the patient's or society's. The concept of utility is discussed in detail in Chapter 3.

$$\text{Cost-Utility Ratio} = \frac{\text{Change in Cost}}{\text{Change in Utility}}$$

A common approach used for employing health utility measures is quality adjusted life years (QALYs), which summarize health utility measures over time. QALYs are a measure of both the quantity and quality of life and are further described in Chapter 3. In such an analysis, the results of the CUA are reported in cost per QALYs gained. Using QALYs in CUA is a common methodology employed by the National Institute for Clinical Excellence (NICE) in the United Kingdom to determine the cost-effectiveness of an intervention. Because the same denominator (QALYs) is used in many economic evaluations, it allows for evaluation of resource allocation across all therapy areas as well as comparison of treatments for a single disease that affects both morbidity and mortality.

An example of CUA is a study by Stein and associates that used a CUA for screening hepatitis C virus (HCV) infection in people attending genitor-urinary medicine (GUM) clinics in the United Kingdom.[9] Cost utility was estimated using an epidemiological model of screening and diagnosis, combined with a Markov chain model of treatment with combination therapy. Literature reviews, expert opinion, and a survey of current screening practice provided parameters for the model. Stein and associates reported the **base case** estimate to be about £85,000 (US $155,379). While the costs were reported as 2001 British pounds (£), the transition to dollars accounted for a more recent exchange rate and not for inflation—in theory both should be taken into consideration. Cost utility for screening restricted to only 20 percent or 10 percent of attendees was estimated as £39,647 (US $72,474.70) and £34,288 (US $62,678.40) per QALY. If screening were restricted only to those with a history of injecting drug use, cost utility would be £27,138 (US $49,608.20) per QALY. Stein and associates concluded that universal screening for HCV in GUM clinics is unlikely to be cost-effective.[9] The methods used by Stein and colleagues also followed the recommendation in the United Kingdom of using a 6 percent discount rate, implying less importance for future costs and QALYs in comparison with the 3 percent recommendation in the United States. In the United States, ICERs of less than $100,000/QALY gained are generally considered cost-effective although there is not universal agreement on the appropriateness of the threshold.

Cost-Benefit Analysis

Cost-benefit analysis (CBA) is a form of economic evaluation in which both the incremental cost and benefits of the intervention are measured in monetary units. The results of the analysis are presented in the form of a **net benefit** (and sometimes the net benefit per dollar spent from a constrained source). The net benefit is simply the difference between the costs and benefits. When the net benefit is positive, the program should be considered economically favorable when considering implementation. Alternatively, a negative net benefit indicates that the intervention costs more than the benefit it yields. The ratio of net benefit per constrained dollar spent helps to rank programs when multiple alternatives can be implemented at once given the resources available. Ranking on the ratio of net benefit, rather than benefit—to constrained dollar spent allows net benefit maximization—the economic objective.

$$\text{Net Benefit to Cost Ratio} = \frac{\text{Net Benefit of Intervention}}{\begin{array}{c}\text{Constrained Dollar}\\\text{Cost of Intervention}\end{array}}$$

To interpret this a bit more, the "constrained dollar cost of the intervention" could be the portion of the cost that is coming from the level of government that is making a decision about implementing a program. When conducting a societal CBA, the total costs could be from a variety of sources other than simply the government. We are interested only in the constrained dollar cost because we are maximizing net benefit per dollar spent by the government (or other decision maker) in order to maximize net benefit for society. Although distributional issues receive some consideration, in general, CBAs are interested in whether there is a positive net benefit regardless of the distribution of costs and benefits.

Because the outcome measures included in CBAs are expressed as a monetary value, the net benefit measure can be used to simply indicate whether one alternative is better than another. This is not possible with CEAs or cost-utility analyses.

One of the limitations of CBA is the method and acceptability of assigning a monetary value (positive or negative) to clinical, QOL, and mortality outcomes. Depending on the methods used to assign these values, they may seem subjective, they may give higher value to wealthier or more highly educated individuals, and they may not agree with local cultural values. In addition, determining which costs to include, particularly for indirect costs, can be controversial. There are also questions concerning whether it is ethical to place different monetary values on individuals who earn different amounts at their jobs.

One example of CBA is a study by Nichol and associates that used a cost-benefit approach from the societal perspective to determine the economic value of influenza vaccination among healthy adults.[10] The basic cost model they employed was:

$$\text{Net Costs (savings)} = C_V - C_{AV}$$

where CV = costs of vaccination and CAV = costs averted due to vaccination

> The cost of vaccination included the direct costs of vaccination (vaccine and its administration), indirect costs associated with lost work time for vaccination, direct costs for potential side effects based on past studies (medical care cost including provider visits, tests, and medication), and indirect cost for lost work time due to potential side effects of vaccination. The cost averted due to vaccination include the direct costs of medical care avoided (healthcare provider visits including test and medication) as well as indirect costs avoided due to work loss and impaired work productivity that were prevented.

The main results are presented in Table 2-3. Nichols and associates estimated vaccination in healthy adults to result in a cost savings of $46.84 per person.[10]

Table 2-3 Economic Benefits Associated with Vaccination

Outcome Variable	Savings (Costs) per 100 Subjects (1994 Dollars)
Direct costs	
Vaccination ($10 per vaccination)*	(1,000.00)
Medical care for side effects (1 office visit per 100 subjects)†‡	(69.51)
Medical care avoided (24 office visits for upper respiratory illness per 100 subjects)†§	1,668.24
Total direct savings	*598.73*
Indirect costs	
Work time lost for vaccination (30 min per vaccination = 50 hours per 100 subjects)* ¶	(583.75)
Work loss due to side effects (2 days per 100 subjects)‡¶	(186.80)
Work loss avoided (52 days for upper respiratory illness per 100 subjects)§¶	4,856.80
Total indirect savings	*4,086.25*
Net savings	**4,684.98**

*A single vaccination was estimated to take 30 minutes of work time and to cost $10, on the basis of a survey of public influenza-vaccination clinics and a local work-site vaccination program.

†A visit to a physician's office, including diagnostic tests and medications, was estimated to cost $69.51.

‡Given the observed though statistically nonsignificant differences between vaccine and placebo recipients, side effects of the vaccine were estimated to result in an additional 2 days of sick leave per 100 subjects vaccinated, with half of these (1 per 100) resulting in a visit to a physician.

§The numbers of days of sick leave and visits to physicians' offices that were avoided are from Table 2-2.

¶Costs of work lost were estimated at $93.40 per day, on the basis of the 1994 median weekly earnings ($467) of full-time U.S. workers.

Source: Nichol, KL, Lind A, et al. The effectiveness of vaccination against influenza in healthy, working adults. *N Engl J Med.* 1995;2333(14)889–893. Copyright © Massachusetts Medical Society. All rights reserved.

Cost of Illness and Burden of Illness Analyses

Cost of illness and burden of illness analyses are not methods of economic evaluation per se, because they involve measuring the costs of a particular disease or illness without consideration of outcome. A **cost of illness** study is defined as an analysis of the total incident lifetime costs (direct and indirect) incurred by a population who come down with a specific disease or condition in a year, while **burden of illness** takes into account the burden due to morbidity and mortality of that specific disease or condition during that year (1998).[11] Cost or burden of illness calculations are tools to assess what types of resources are consumed and how much these resources cost, individually and in aggregate to the system (and has been proposed as one method to ascertain levels of research funding). For instance, in the study by Weiss and associates, they estimate the annual costs of managing asthma in the United States were estimated to be $10.7 billion, approximating $6.1 billion in direct costs and $4.6 billion in indirect costs (more on direct and indirect costs later). Of the $6.1 billion in direct costs, emergency department visits accounted for 8 percent, hospitalizations for 29 percent, outpatient hospital costs for 10 percent, physician services for 12 percent, and medications for 40 percent.[12]

Use of Models in Conducting Formal Economics Assessments

Modeling is an analytical and/or visual tool that represents a hypothetical situation or system of interest. There are several types of models that can be used in economic evaluation of healthcare interventions. Models are useful for predicting future costs and outcomes associated with two or more medical treatments and are often used to answer a question that would normally be difficult to answer due to time restraints, financial barriers, or lack of complete empiric data. Although modeling cannot be done without any empiric data, it can be created when a particular piece or combination of data is not available. Examples of data sources used in economic modeling are provided in Figure 2-4. Hospital, physician, or other providers' charges for medical services should not be used as data sources for economic models, because these figures are considered to be inaccurate measures of cost. Actual costs may be available from healthcare providers, depending on the sophistication of their accounting system. Alternatively, actual costs may be estimated by summing the resources used (such as supplies, labor, and facility overhead) or by multiplying charges by an acceptable cost-to-charge ratio.

Figure 2-4 Sources of Data Used in Economic Models

Sources of data on the intervention(s) outcomes	Sources of data on the intervention(s) costs

1. Medical literature
2. Datasets
   a. National
   b. Commercial
3. Expert opinion (last resort)
	1. Reimbursement rates
	2. Hospital, health plan, CMS
	3. Red book (average wholesale price for drugs)
	4. Actual costs (may be available, depending on the sophistication of the accounting system)
	5. May also be calculated, by estimating cost of care based on resource use

Decision Analysis

One of the more widely accepted modeling methods is **decision analysis**. This method is defined as an explicit, quantitative, and systematic approach to decision making under conditions of uncertainty in which probabilities of each possible event, along with the consequence of those events, are stated.[13] One of the advantages of decision analysis is that it is transparent. However, its usefulness may be limited by the outcome measures selected and/or the quality of data available to populate the model.

Decision trees are often used to graphically illustrate decision analyses (Figure 2-5). A basic decision tree figure is made up of branches and nodes. The first node that makes up the tree is called the **decision node** (square). This is where all the choices facing the decision maker is stated and where the branches of each treatment arm originate. The treatment arms then branch out to represent different outcomes. The node where the outcome branches originate is called a **chance node** (circle). These next nodes represent all outcomes for a single event and are assigned probabilities for that particular outcome. Each branch of the decision tree must be mutually exclusive. In addition, each node (where the branches converge) should equal the sum of probabilities assigned to each converging branch. Finally, after all outcomes are exhausted, each branch ends with a **terminal node** (triangle). Each terminal node is assigned a cost or value called a **payoff**. For example, Figure 5-2 presents with two treatment arms (treatment arm 1 and treatment arm 2). Each treatment arm has two mutually exclusive outcomes associated with different payoffs (terminal nodes).

The steps required to perform a decision analysis are summarized in Figure 2-6. First, the relevant interventions are identified. The framework of the decision tree is then constructed, and the probability of each outcome occurring is assigned (p1, p2, p3, and p4). The value of each of these outcomes is then applied to each branch (v1, v2, v3, and v4). Values are typically expressed in monetary

Figure 2-5 Basic Decision Tree Structure

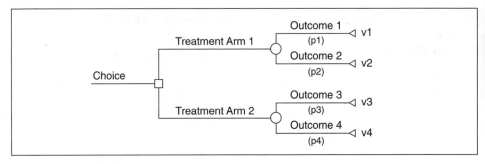

units (when the total cost of competing interventions is of interest) or in utilities (when patients' utility for competing interventions is of interest). Finally, the **expected value** of each arm is calculated as the sum of probabilities multiplied by outcomes values, as follows:

$$\text{Treatment Arm 1} = (p1)(v1) + (p2)(v2)$$
$$\text{Treatment Arm 2} = (p3)(v3) + (p4)(v4)$$

A **sensitivity analysis** (discussed in Chapter 5) is then performed to test the robustness of the model.

An example of a decision tree can be found in study by Goldfarb and associates. In this study, the standard procedure in diagnosing Crohn's disease was compared to a new technology known as wireless capsule endoscopy.[4] Medicare reimbursement fees (2003) were used to represent the costs, while pooled diagnostic yields and probabilities of complications during the diagnostic procedure were used to populate the model (Figure 2-7).

The cost associated with wireless capsule endoscopy was $1547 compared to $1838 using the standard diagnostic procedure (small bowel follow-through and colonoscopy). Therefore, the economic analysis concluded that, from a payer's perspective, wireless capsule endoscopy would most likely be less costly than current diagnostic practice.

Figure 2-6 Steps in Performing a Decision Analysis

1. Identify the decision and relevant treatment alternatives.
2. Structure the decision tree and the consequences of each decision.
3. Assess the probabilities of each consequence.
4. Value outcomes (using either cost or utility as the outcome measure).
5. Calculate the expected value of each decision.
6. Determine the robustness of the model using sensitivity analyses.
7. Choose the preferred course of action.

Figure 2-7 Decision Tree for the Diagnosis of Crohn's Disease

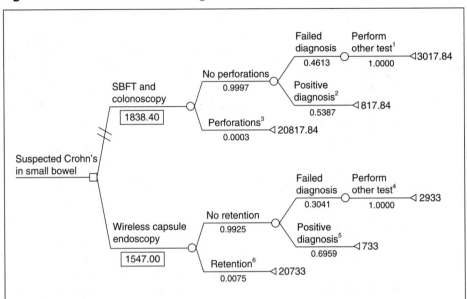

Estimated costs for "other test," derived from the Hay study and adjusted to 2003 USD, was $2200. Medicare costs for SFBT and colonoscopy were $817.84. Medicare costs for WCE were $733.00. Costs for perforations and retention were estimated to be $20,000.

[1]Total cost of other tests plus Medicare cost for SBFT and colonoscopy
[2]Total cost for positive test from SBFT and colonoscopy
[3]Total cost for perforations and Medicare cost for SBFT and colonoscopy
[4]Total cost of other tests plus Medicare cost for WCE
[5]Total cost for positive test from WCE
[6]Total cost for perforations and Medicare cost for WCE

Source: Disease Management Winter 2004. Reprinted with permission from *Disease Management*, published by Mary Ann Liebert, Inc. New Rochelle, NY.

Budget Impact Models

One of the simpler types of models is a **budget impact model** (BIM). BIMs, or cost-impact analyses, are used to predict the budgetary impact of a new intervention or a change in utilization patterns for existing treatments. In its strictest form, BIM assumes that outcomes of two or more modeled interventions are equal (as a CMA). In addition, some BIMs may consider cost savings due to improved outcomes, such as reduced length of stay, emergency department admissions, or physician visits.

Other Types of Models

More elaborate models in economic evaluation are Markov models and Monte Carlo simulations. **Markov models** are used to capture the changes in disease states that can reoccur over time (such as movement between progression or remission of disease) or treatment algorithms that are cyclical in design. Markov models can be understood as a type of repetitive decision tree.[14] A **Monte Carlo simulation** is a method of repeating the model over a range of possible probabilities and combinations of inputs. Like most models, the treatment population must be specified and the assumptions defined.

Evaluating the Quality of Economics Assessments

Although there is a growing body of health economic literature, the validity and reliability of these studies can range greatly. Therefore, standards or guidelines need to be established in order to assess the quality of these studies and to determine which studies would weigh more when making healthcare decisions. There are various evaluation tools that can be found in the literature. One example is the Quality of Health Economic Studies (QHES) instrument developed by Ofman and colleagues.[15] The QHES (Figure 2-8) provides a list of 16 items that should be checked in evaluating a CEA. It is difficult to give a quantitative assessment to the value of each item. Instead, the combination of items that follow and the ability to follow recommendations should be carefully considered when evaluating the quality of a study.

Conclusion

High-quality economic analyses can be an important tool in making resource allocation decisions that will help to control the ever-increasing costs in health care. Although they have not necessarily been used much in making policy in the United States to date, the continued development of methods for analysis and presentation of the results will make them easier to use as the importance of more rational resource allocation continues to become more apparent to healthcare policy makers and patients.

This chapter presented with a brief overview of the tools and methods needed to measure economic outcomes. Before conducting any economic analyses, a clear understanding of the appropriate types of costs must first be established. Therefore, it is important to be able to distinguish between direct, indirect, and intangible cost. A useful visualization tool to organize various cost factors is an Ishikawa diagram. Economic assessments incorporate various forms of costs,

Figure 2-8 Questions for Assessing the Value and Quality of Health Economic Information

1. Was the study objective presented in a clear, specific, and measurable manner?
2. Were the perspective of the analysis (societal, third-party payer, etc.) and reasons for its selection stated?
3. Were variable estimates used in the analysis from the best available source (i.e., Randomized Controlled Trial-Best, Expert Opinion-Worst)?
4. If estimates came from a subgroup analysis, were the groups prespecified at the beginning of the study?
5. Was uncertainty handled by (1) statistical analysis to address random events or (2) sensitivity analysis to cover a range of assumptions?
6. Was incremental analysis performed between alternatives for resources and costs?
7. Was the methodology for data abstraction (including the value of health states and other benefits) stated?
8. Did the analytic horizon allow time for all relevant and important outcomes? Were benefits and costs that went beyond 1 year discounted (3–5%) and justification given for the discount rate?
9. Was the measurement of costs appropriate and the methodology for the estimation of quantities and unit costs clearly described?
10. Were the primary outcome measure(s) for the economic evaluation clearly stated and did they include the major short-term, long-term, and negative outcomes?
11. Were the health outcome(s) measures/scales valid and reliable? If previously tested valid and reliable measures were not available, was justification given for the measures/scales used?
12. Were the economic model (including structure), study methods and analysis, and the components of the numerator and denominator displayed in a clear, transparent manner?
13. Were the choice of economic model, main assumptions, and limitation of the study stated and justified?
14. Did the author(s) explicitly discuss direction and magnitude of potential biases?
15. Were the conclusion/recommendations of the study justified and based on the study results?
16. Was there a statement disclosing the source of funding for the study?

Source: Adapted and reprinted with permission from the *Journal of Managed Care Pharmacy.* Ofman JJ, Sullivan SD, Neumann PJ, et al. Examining the value and quality of health economic analyses: Implication of utlizing the QHES. *J Manag Care Pharm.* 2003;9(1):53–61.

both direct and indirect, with specific outcomes and quantify the results into comparable means. There are also various methods to conduct economic assessments that range in techniques (CMA, CCA, CEA, CUA, and CBA). Understanding the difference and appropriateness of each method is crucial. Modeling then completes the picture by applying these methods to specific research questions. For example, they are useful for predicting future costs and outcomes associated with two or more medical treatments.

By learning the tools and techniques used in measuring economic outcomes, one can conduct and evaluate economic studies used in decision making and therefore can understand and participate in important and complex economic decisions affecting health care today.

■ Case Study

As medical director at CareWell, you are leading the development of a clinical practice guideline for major depressive disorder (MDD; e.g., depression). You have narrowed your selection of the first-line antidepressant medication to one of two drugs—Happynol or Moodlift. Before selecting one of these medications for the guideline, you would like to evaluate the cost-effectiveness of the two options using decision analysis. As a health plan, CareWell is concerned with managing only the direct medical costs of treatment.

As you set forth to build your tree, you gather the following information:

Happynol is 90 percent effective in the treatment of MDD. However, over a 3-month period of use, 20 percent of patients develop severe adverse events. Half of the patients (50 percent) who develop an adverse event will discontinue the medication and need to be switched to an alternative medication. Moodlift is 80 percent effective for the treatment of MDD and has a 5 percent incidence of mild adverse events over a 3-month period; 10 percent of patients who experience such events will discontinue their medication and need to be switched to an alternative medication. All effectively treated patients adhere to their medication schedule; all patients who do not experience treatment effectiveness discontinue their medication at the end of 3 months and need to be switched to an alternative medication. A 3-month treatment with Happynol costs CareWell $200. The same treatment with Moodlift costs CareWell $300. Because both drugs are dispensed in 90-day supplies, the cost of drug is the same for patients who adhere for a full three months and patients who discontinue their drug and are switched at some point during the three months. The average cost of an adverse event with Happynol is $1200, while an adverse event due to Moodlift costs $100. The cost of switching medications, due to nonadherence, adverse events, and/or ineffectiveness, for either medication, is $150, which results from additional follow-up care for reevaluation of therapy and selection of an alternative antidepressant medication. Assume all other costs, for example, the cost of routine physician visits, are the same for both groups.

You construct a decision tree based on the previous scenario (Case Figure 2-1).

Next, you calculate the total cost of treating a patient with Happynol versus Moodlift by "folding" or "rolling back" each arm of the tree (Case Figure 2-2).

Case Figure 2-1 Decision Tree Depicting the Treatment Alternatives

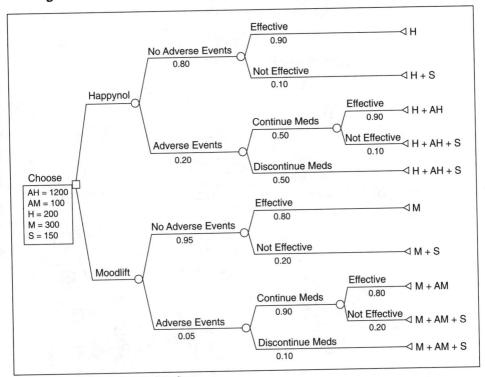

Note: This tree is constructed using the TreeAge Data software.

Key
AH—Cost of an Adverse Event with Happynol ($1200)
AM—Cost of an Adverse Event with Moodlife ($100)
H—Cost of Happynol ($200)
M—Cost of Moodlift ($300)
S—Cost of switching meds for either medication ($150)

Case Figure 2-2   Decision Tree with Costs Included

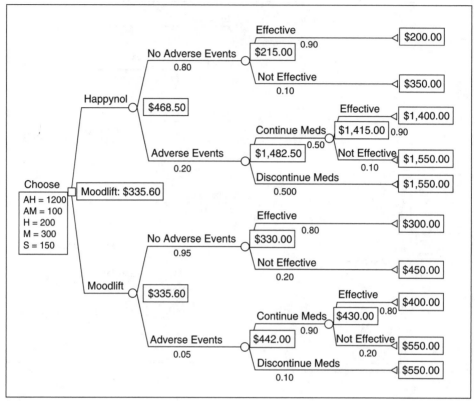

Note: Calculations performed using TreeAge Data software.

Key
AH—Cost of an Adverse Event with Happynol ($1200)
AM—Cost of an Adverse Event with Moodlife ($100)
H—Cost of Happynol ($200)
M—Cost of Moodlift ($300)
S—Cost of switching meds for either medication ($150)

Based on the lower total cost ($335.60), you choose Moodlift.

Study/Discussion Questions

1. What are the similarities and differences between the various types of formal economic analyses? What are the advantages and disadvantages of each?
2. What are direct and indirect costs? Provide examples of each.
3. What is modeling? What is decision analysis and when is this technique useful? What are some potential data sources used in economic models?

Suggested Readings/Web Sites

Bureau of Labor Statistics. Available at: www.bls.org.

International Society for Pharmoeconomics and Outcomes Research. Available at: www.ispor.org.

Drummond MF, O'Brian BJ, Stoddart GL, Torrance GW. *Methods for the Economic Evaluation of Health Care Programmes*. 2nd ed. New York: Oxford University Press; 1997.

Gold M, Siegel J, Russell L, Weinstein M. *Cost Effectiveness in Health and Medicine*. New York: Oxford University Press; 1996.

References

1. Drummond MF, O'Brien BJ, Stoddart GL, Torrance GW. *Methods for the Economic Evaluation of Health Care Programmes*. 2nd ed. New York: Oxford University Press; 1997.
2. Finkler SA. The distinction between costs and charges. *Ann Intern Med*. 1982; 96(1):102–109.
3. Paddock LE, Phillips AC. Quality improvement tools in disease management. *Dis Manag*. 2001;4(2):1–10.
4. Goldfarb NI, Pizzi LT, Fuhr JP Jr, et al. Diagnosing Crohn's disease: an economic analysis comparing wireless capsule endoscopy with traditional diagnostic procedures. (Review) *Dis Manag*. 2004;7(4):292–304.
5. Gold M, Siegel J, Russell L, Winstein M. *Cost Effectiveness in Health and Medicine*. New York: Oxford University Press; 1996.
6. Chen GJ, Ferrucci L, Moran WP, Pahor M. A cost-minimization analysis of diuretic-based antihypertensive therapy reducing cardiovascular events in older adults with isolated systolic hypertension. *Cost Eff Resour Alloc*. 2005;3(1):2.
7. Mauskopf JA, Paul JE, Grant DM, Stergachis A. The role of cost-consequence analysis in healthcare decision making. *Pharmacoeconomics*. 1998;13(3):277–288.
8. Khandker RK, Dulski JD, Kilpatrick JB, Ellis RP, Mitchell JB, Baine WB. A decision model and cost-effectiveness analysis of colorectal cancer screening and surveillance guidelines for average-risk adults. *Int J Technol Assess Health Care*. 2000;16(3):799–810.

9. Stein K, Dalzeil K, Walker A, Jenkins B, Round A, Royle P. Screening for hepatitis C in genitor-urinary medicine clinics: A cost utility analysis. *J Hepatol.* 2003;39(5):814–825.

10. Nichol KL, Lind A, Margolis KL et al. The effectiveness of vaccination against influenza in healthy, working adults. *N Engl J Med.* 1995;333(14):889–893.

11. Wiseman V, Mooney G. Burden of illness estimates for priority setting: a debate revisited. *Health Policy.* 1998;43(3):243–251.

12. Weiss KB, Sullivan SD, Lyttle CS. Trends in the cost of illness for asthma in the United States, 1985–1994. *J Allergy Clin Immunol.* 2000;106(3):493–499.

13. Sox HC. Decision analysis: A basic clinical skill? *N Engl J Med.* 1987;316(5):271–272.

14. Stokey E, Zeckhauer R. A *Primer for Policy Analysis.* New York: Norton and Co.; 1978.

15. Ofman JJ, Sullivan SD, Neumann PJ et al. Examining the value and quality of health economic analyses; Implication of utilizing the QHES. *J Manag Care Pharm.* 2003;9(1): 53–61.

Chapter 3

HEALTH-RELATED QUALITY OF LIFE AND HEALTH UTILITY

Christine Weston, MSEd, PhD
Dong-Churl Suh, MBA, PhD

Overview

This chapter is about measuring health-related quality of life and health utility, both of which may be used in economic evaluation. Quality-of-life assessment allows us to identify the burden of illness experienced by patients and to compare the effectiveness of medical treatments. This information is useful not only to doctors and their patients, but to decision makers who are responsible for evaluating the costs and effectiveness of healthcare interventions. There are typically two different ways to measure health-related quality of life, arising from two different disciplines. The first is health-status assessment, from the field of psychometrics; the second is patient-preference assessment, from the science of econometrics. There are advantages and disadvantages to both approaches, but each has an important role in evaluating the effectiveness of healthcare interventions. In measuring health-related quality of life, a patient is asked to provide responses to a series of questions about their subjective well-being. These measures allow us to compare groups of patients receiving different treatments or to identify change over time in the same group of patients. On the other hand, preference-based utility measures reflect the value of certain health states to an individual under conditions of uncertainty. Patient-preference assessment is primarily used to determine the trade-off between the quality and quantity of life. This chapter provides an in-depth view of quality of life and the use of utilities in calculating quality adjusted life years for cost-effectiveness analyses and other economic evaluations.

Learning Objectives

1. To become familiar with terminology related to quality of life and be able to distinguish between quality of life and health-related quality of life
2. To understand how quality of life research has evolved over the last decade
3. To recognize the multiple purposes for measuring quality of life
4. To learn the difference between generic and disease-specific instruments
5. To become familiarized with the methodological and measurement issues in QOL research
6. To understand the concept of health utility and the three major methods used to estimate it
7. To understand the quality adjusted life years (QALY) measure and how it is used in economic evaluation

Keywords

Cardinal utilities
European Quality of Life Index
Expected utility theory
Health utilities index
Health-related quality of life
Humanistic outcomes
Medical outcomes study
Ordinal utilities
Patient-centered outcomes
Patient-reported outcomes
Patient satisfaction
Preferences
Quality of life
Quality of Well-Being Scale
Quality adjusted life years
Rating scale technique
SF-36
SF-6D
Standard gamble technique
Time trade-off method
Utility

Introduction

Although clinical measures are the most common outcomes assessed in scientific research of healthcare interventions, over the past 10 to 15 years growing recognition has been paid to the importance of humanistic outcomes. **Humanistic outcomes** are measures that put primary emphasis on the *patient's* perception of their health status and health outcomes. Examples of humanistic end points include quality of life, health status, and functional well-being.

This shift in emphasis from objective clinical measures to a focus on the patient's subjective experience coincides with a change in emphasis in modern medicine from the diagnosis and cure of infectious disease to a preoccupation with chronic disease. This change has led to an increased focus on collecting patient-reported outcomes in order to understand the impact of treatment on patient functioning and well-being. This information is important not only to physicians and their patients, but to key decision makers, including policy makers, regulatory agencies, managed care organizations, and payers.

Quality of life is a concept that has received increased attention over the last few decades and its importance is only beginning to be realized in the actual practice of clinical medicine. The concept that was virtually absent in medical research until the 1970s, is now considered to be an important measure by current standards. Formal acknowledgment of this perspective is exemplified by the emergence of the term *patient-reported outcomes* in clinical trial research.[1, 2, 3] One example of this change in emphasis can be observed in studies of migraine headache. Traditional endpoints of migraine would include changes in numerical indices of the intensity, duration, and frequency of attacks. However, new guidelines recommend that the essential aim of migraine treatments should be to reduce the global impact of the headaches on the patient's life.[4] Another example is related to current research in the area of attention deficit hyperactivity disorder (ADHD). The traditional aim of treatment in this field would usually be focused on symptom reduction, but current aims encompass a wider view that takes into account the overall health-related quality of life of children and adolescents, as well as their families whose lives are also affected by the disorder.[5]

Another major factor for the increased focus on quality-of-life research has to do with the undesirable side effects of many modern treatments. Although treatment advances may extend years of life, they may also seriously compromise the *quality* of a patient's life. Understanding patients' perspectives on these issues is vital to offering them the interventions that are best suited for their needs and desires. Furthermore, growing evidence demonstrates that some diseases or conditions can lead to greater emotional rather than physical suffering. Therefore, failure to measure the social and emotional effects of illness provides only a partial picture of its impact on patients.

Finally, there is increasing recognition that changes in quality of life do not necessarily coincide with physiologic changes. On the one hand, some studies have shown that there can be changes in functional status without evidence of physiologic improvement. Conversely, physiologic improvement may occur without discernible clinical benefits. This point also supports the need for end points that extend beyond clinical measures.

■ Defining Quality of Life

Quality of life (QOL) and **health-related quality of life** (HR-QOL) are terms that are often used interchangeably. Healthcare researchers often say "quality of life" for short when what they really mean is "health-related quality of life." It is important to understand the distinction between the two concepts. Quality of life is a broad concept that refers to an individual's overall assessment of their quality of life. This can include social, emotional, spiritual, health, financial, and various other domains of life; health-related quality of life refers to an assessment of those aspects of life that pertain specifically to health status or health outcomes.

The term *humanistic outcomes* refers to outcomes that concern the impact of a disease or condition on an *individual*, as opposed to outcomes that are exclusively clinical or economic. However, it is a more inclusive term than quality of life because it includes other measures of health status, patient satisfaction, work outcomes, and patient-based assessments. Humanistic outcomes include any measure concerning the patient's perspective. For example, one could measure the *clinical effects* of a treatment for asthma, study the *direct costs* of a treatment for asthma, or one could examine the impact of the treatment on *humanistic outcomes*: How does this treatment affect the patient's QOL, their ability to function, to socialize, to travel, to be productive at work? All of these questions relate to the humanistic impact of the treatment.

A more recently coined phrase that overlaps with the concept of HR-QOL is **patient-reported outcomes** (PROs). This term has become more popular in recent years because patient-reported outcomes have become important primary or secondary end points in clinical trial research.[6] As aptly explained by Wiklund,[7]

> As the patient is the primary recipient of treatment, there is a need to recognize and value the patient's perception of change in response to treatment in clinical trials.

PROs generally include measures of subjective symptoms, HR-QOL, and treatment satisfaction. **Patient-centered outcomes** is a synonymous, but less widely used term.

PROs are based on a patient's assessment of the effect of a treatment or therapy, which may indeed be different than what can be directly observed or measured by a clinician. In some cases, PROs may, in fact, be a better indication of the impact of the treatment. As an example, a recent study compared patient and physician reported outcomes of a treatment for patients with rheumatoid arthritis.[8] The patient-reported measures included a self-assessment of pain, a global health assessment, and measure of physical function; physician-reported measures included tender and swollen joint counts, a physician global assessment, and the results of laboratory tests. Result of this study demonstrated a better discrimination of treatment effect with PROs compared to physician-reported outcomes.

A separate, but related, area of study is **patient satisfaction** with healthcare services, which can be defined as the extent of an individual's experience compared with his or her expectations.[8] Although some may regard patient satisfaction as a relatively unimportant outcome or end point, satisfaction may be clinically important because satisfied patients are more likely to comply with treatment, to take an active role in their own health care, to continue using medical services, and to stay with a provider. The end result is that patients who are satisfied are more likely to have better health outcomes. One drawback of patient satisfaction is that there are far fewer standard approaches to measuring patient satisfaction compared to QOL.

Conceptual Description of QOL

QOL has been defined in numerous ways by countless numbers of researchers; consequently there is no universally accepted conceptual construct. Nevertheless, it is generally accepted that the concept of QOL is one that is both *multidimensional* and *subjective*.[9, 10, 11, 12] QOL is multidimensional because it encompasses an individual's global evaluation of their physical, emotional, and social well-being. It reflects how people feel, and their ability to function in their everyday life. QOL is subjective because it refers to an individual's subjective sense of well-being, as opposed to objective circumstances. Although it is generally understood that objective conditions or circumstances (such as health, wealth, and comfort) may influence subjective well-being, they are do not adequately reflect the concept implied by QOL.

Our current-day understanding of QOL has probably been influenced in great part by the World Health Organization's (WHO) definitions of both health and QOL, specifically because these definitions reflect a view of health that extends far beyond physical illness. WHO's definition of health is "a state of complete physical, mental, and social well-being and not merely the absence of disease or infirmity." The WHO definition of QOL is "an individual's perceptions of their position in life in the context of the culture and value system in which they live and in relation to their goals, standards, and concerns."[11, 12, 13]

According to Spilker, QOL is generally measured by three interrelated levels that build on each other.[11] At the top of the pyramid is an overall assessment of well-being; immediately following are the broad domains that contribute to the global sense of well-being (i.e., physical, psychological, economic, spiritual, social); and at the bottom are the components of each domain.

How Has QOL Research Evolved?

The importance and popularity of HR-QOL has been expanding steadily over the past several decades. A search of two databases—Ovid MEDLINE and the Cochrane Central Register of Controlled Trials—for publications including the term *quality of life* reveals just how much research has increased over the past 30 years. From 1970 to 1979, there were only 350 QOL publications indexed in the MEDLINE database. This number increased by five times that amount in the 1980s, and in the 1990s, increased by almost five times again. Most impressive is what has occurred since 2000. From then to 2005, there were 8645 references with the subject heading QOL—a number greater than the total number of articles published during the entire last decade. The use of QOL data in controlled trials (such as the Cochrane Central Register) has also ballooned during the past 10 years, with the inclusion of QOL as a measure in randomized controlled trials increasing from a mere 31 studies in the 1970s to over 3400 during the last four years.

Why Measure Quality of Life?

There are multiple purposes for measuring QOL. The first, and perhaps the most common use of QOL data, is to assess the burden of illness on patients, their families, and society as a whole. Assessment of QOL allows us to understand to what extent a given disease or condition:

Figure 3-1 Dimensions of Quality of Life

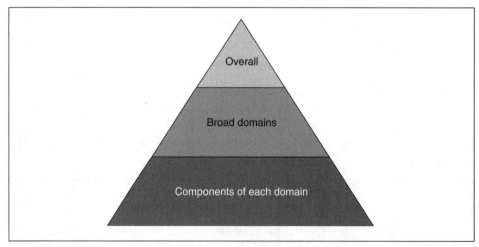

Source: Spilker, B (ed). *Quality of Life and Pharmacoeconomics in Clinical Trials.* Second Edition. Philadelphia: Lippincott-Raven, 1996.[11]

Table 3-1 Number of Quality of Life Publications, 1970–Present

Time Period	Ovid MEDLINE **# of references**	Cochrane Central Register of Controlled Trials **# of references**
1970–1979	350	31
1980–1989	1738	306
1990–1999	8107	3546
2000–2005	8645	3415

- Deteriorates emotional well-being
- Interferes with the ability to participate in social and leisure activities
- Disrupts family relationships
- Causes disability, absenteeism, or a decline in productivity at work
- Leads to caregiver burden

Consider this example. Prescription medications have had a significant impact on the lives of people with HIV/AIDS. Studies that measure the QOL of these individuals can provide a wealth of information to doctors, patients, researchers, and health policy makers. Studies have been conducted that allow researchers to examine the relationship between traditional variables, such as patient survival and cost of care and QOL. One study examined the QOL of people living with AIDS in 1984 to those in 1998, and found that patients in the latter cohort had lower costs as well as better quality of life.[14] Another study found that the while the cost of drug treatment is high, people with better treatment were able to return to work, which had a significantly positive impact on their self-reported QOL.[15]

Another major purpose for measuring QOL is to determine the effectiveness of medical treatments. QOL not only allows us to understand the value of specific medical therapies, but allows us to *compare* the relative merits of different healthcare interventions. As an example, current options for the treatment of prostate cancer include radical prostatectomy, cryosurgery, radiotherapy, hormone therapy, and watchful waiting.[16] Many of the long-term effects of treatment can have a large impact on patients' QOL, and in some patients, may offset the clinical benefits. This is precisely where inclusion of QOL data can be useful in helping to determine the best choice of treatment for patients.

QOL end points are studied for another reason. To put it simply, in some situations, QOL may actually be a better indicator of health than traditional clinical measures—particularly for diseases and conditions in which diagnosis relies more heavily on patient-reported symptoms than on clinical symptomatology.

One example of this is gastro-esophageal reflux disease (GERD). Although tests are available, patients often report symptoms of heartburn and reflux, despite negative endoscopies. In this situation, if physicians were to rely exclusively on clinical tests to the neglect of patient-reported symptoms, an accurate assessment of treatment would be obscured.[17]

A similar example concerns patients with end-stage renal disease. One study found that patients' scores on the physical component of the Kidney Disease Quality of Life Short Form (KDQOL-SF) were more accurate in identifying patients at risk for death than serum albumin levels, and that in general, HR-QOL played an important role in predicting adverse events in patients with end-stage renal disease.[18]

QOL measurement is particularly relevant for patients with cancer.[8, 12] Traditional cancer outcomes are length of disease-free survival, relapse rates, disease progression, or tumor response, yet sorely missing is the way that treatment affects the QOL of cancer patients. When QOL is included in cancer clinical trials, it can provide physicians and patients with information that can help them identify better treatments. QOL outcomes are now a major component of cancer clinical trials, as well as other trials. Additionally, QOL end points are recent adjuncts to studies on treatment cost-effectiveness and survival analysis. Consequently QOL research is considered by many a fundamental task of oncology research.[2]

Measuring Quality of Life

What Are the Different Types of Quality of Life Instruments?

In general, QOL instruments vary along three different continuums: generic versus disease-specific measures, single-dimension versus broad-spectrum measures, and the type of values resulting from the measure. Some instruments are designed to assess the HR-QOL related to a specific disease or condition, while others are generic (e.g., applicable to a broad range of diseases and conditions). It is important to realize that there is no one perfect measure and each has its own costs and benefits. Some of the benefits of disease-specific measures are that they have greater meaning to physicians, they are able to focus on particular areas of concern, and they may possess greater responsiveness to disease-specific interventions. Proponents of disease-specific measures say that they are "useful in clinical trials and practice because they are more responsive to small but clinically important changes than generic instruments." On the other hand, generic measures are particularly useful for comparisons across diagnostic conditions or interventions. Generic instruments are best for estimating the burden of illness experienced by a group of patients with one condition compared to the burden experienced by patients with another condition; for example, how QOL of patients with migraine compare to QOL of asthmatics.

Generic Instruments

Though there are several established generic HR-QOL instruments, the most well-known and widely used generic health survey is the **Medical Outcomes Study** Short Form 36 (**SF-36**). There are various forms of the SF health survey, including a newer version, a shorter version, and a version for use with children. However, all of the SF surveys measure the same eight domains of health: physical functioning, role limitations due to physical health (role-physical), bodily pain, general health perceptions, vitality, social functioning, role limitations due to emotional problems (role-emotional), and mental health. Use of the SF-36 yields two types of scores: (1) an individual score for each domain or scale, and (2) a physical and mental component summary score.[19]

In addition to the SF-36, there are a number of other generic QOL instruments. Another, the Dartmouth COOP Functional Health Assessment Charts were developed for the purpose of making a brief, practical, and valid method to assess the functional status of adults and adolescents. The system was developed by the Dartmouth COOP Project, a network of community medical practices that cooperate on primary care research activities. Each chart consists of a title, a question referring to the status of the patient over the past 2–4 weeks, and 5 response choices. This instrument is different from the SF-36 in that question responses are illustrated by a drawing that depicts a level of functioning or well-being. Dimensions of health status measured by the health charts are physical, emotional, daily activities, social activities, social support, pain, and overall health.[20]

The Duke Health Profile (DUKE) is a 17-item generic questionnaire that measures respondent-reported functional health status and HR-QOL during a one-week time period. It is user-friendly, brief, easy to understand, and has only three simple response options. This profile has six scales measure functional health (physical, mental, social, general, perceived health, and self-esteem), and five scales that measure dysfunctional health (anxiety, depression, anxiety-depression, pain, and disability).[21]

The Sickness Impact Profile (SIP) is a 136-item self- or interviewer-administered that health status questionnaire which measures everyday activities according to 12 categories (sleep and rest, emotional behavior, body care and movement, home management, mobility, social interaction, ambulation, alertness behavior, communication, work, recreation and pastimes, and eating). Respondents "endorse" items that describe themselves and are related to their health.[22]

Disease-Specific Instruments

There are also dozens of disease-specific instruments that have been developed for a wide-range of illnesses and medical conditions. One example is the Asthma Quality of Life Questionnaire. This measures uses a 7-point Likert scale to assess symptoms, emotions, exposure to environmental stimuli, and activity limitation. Another, the Diabetes Quality of Life (DQOL) measure was the groundbreaking instrument originally developed for the Diabetes Control and Complications Trial (DCCT) in the early 1980s.[23] Like these, other instruments exist for conditions ranging from ADHD and depression to overactive bladder and pain.

Choosing an Instrument

When designing a study involving QOL measurement, should one choose a generic or disease-specific instrument? This question has been the subject of much debate. The best answer to the question probably is "it depends." The instrument a researcher chooses will depend on the particular disease or condition under study, the goals of the study, the availability of disease-specific measures, and the psychometric soundness of the instruments available. Some researchers have found that disease-specific instruments are superior to generic instruments in predicting functional impairment and QOL, while others suggest that disease-specific measures are poor indicators of overall HR-QOL.[24,25] Perhaps the inclusion of both generic and disease-specific instruments in a particular study is the best way to capture a comprehensive understanding of the QOL impact of the condition.[26,27] It is also important to consider whether your instrument of choice is culturally sensitive to the population of interest. Finally, QOL instruments must be supported by psychometric data that demonstrate reliability (reproducibility), validity, and responsiveness.[13]

Methodological and Measurement Issues

There are many methodological and measurement issues in assessing QOL. One of the most important questions concerns how to assess and interpret changes in QOL over time. Another concerns how to interpret the clinical significance of QOL results. How is statistical significance translated into meaningful change? Other issues concern how to handle multiple QOL outcomes within the same study. An article by Sprangers and associates delineates important questions that may serve as guidelines for assessing and interpreting change.[28] Ultimately, however, the way QOL data are applied to decision making depends on the unique perspective of the stakeholder, as illustrated by the following quote:[29]

> A clinician may attempt to explain to a patient potential treatment alternatives for his or her QOL; a health policymaker may try to describe to elected officials the financial impact on a patient population with reduced QOL; a researcher

may try to obtain the vital messages from a clinical trial that included QOL endpoints; and a regulatory agency and/or pharmaceutical company may try to ascertain the appropriate level of evidence required for a successful research study.

Defining Health Utility

Utility is one of the measures used to value benefits of certain interventions or programs and describe the burden of disease or health outcome in a specific population. The term **utility** was introduced by von Neumann and Morgenstern in 1944 in their theory of rational decision making under uncertainty. This theory is sometimes called the **expected utility theory**, or von Neumann-Morgenstern expected utility theory.[30] Von Neumann and Morgenstern described how a rational individual would make decisions when faced with several uncertain outcomes (e.g., choosing between two lotteries). Generally, utility refers to the **preferences** (or desirability) individuals or society place on any specific outcome (e.g., for a given health state) relative to other possible outcomes. The more preferable the outcome, the more utility is associated with it because utility measures the strength of person's preferences for different outcomes and conditions under uncertainty. Because most health outcomes are uncertain in the real world, defining preferences under uncertainty (utilities) is more applicable than defining preferences under certainty.[31]

Utility in the Context of Economic Evaluation: QALYs

Utility valuation is particularly useful because it allows the calculation of a generic outcome measure called **quality adjusted life years** (QALYs). QALYs are defined as the life years gained by program implementation adjusted for the patient's QOL, including both mortality and morbidity issues and have been cited as the most common used unit for measuring patient QOL. QALYs are commonly used as an outcome measure in economic evaluations, particularly cost-effectiveness and cost-utility analyses. The quality adjustment is based on the application of weights when calculating health expectancy—one for each possible health state that represents the relative desirability of the health state.[31, 32] This enables a broad range of relevant outcomes, such as quantity of life or survival times in health states (mortality) and quality of life (morbidity), to be simultaneously combined into a single composite summary outcome.[31, 33] The number of QALYs assess the period of time in a state of perfect health that the respondent says is equivalent to a period in ill health, and therefore represents the number of healthy years of life that are valued equivalently to the actual health outcome.[33, 34] In addition, QALYs allow broad comparisons across widely differing programs. QALYs are generally calculated by multiplying the time a person stays in each health state by the utility value of that health state and summing up the obtained products for all states.

Measuring Health Utility

Utilities are measured on an ordinal or cardinal scale. **Ordinal utilities** simply rank health states or outcomes in order of their preference.[35] **Cardinal utilities,** which are more commonly used, are a set of numbers assigned to the health states or outcomes such that the number represents the strength of subject's preference for a specific health status relative to the others. Individual subject utilities are assigned using utility instruments, which standardize scores of health status on a scale from 0 (representing death) to 1 (representing perfect health). Utilities can be measured directly or indirectly. The three most widely used approaches to measure utility values directly are the standard gamble, time trade-off, and rating scale approaches.[35] Indirect methods, use of expert judgment, the scientific literature, and generic instruments to obtain utility values are also summarized.

Standard Gamble Technique

The **standard gamble technique** is considered an established method of measuring utility values because of its strong normative foundation in von Neumann-Morgenstern utility theory.[36] Standard gamble technique is a classic method used to measure cardinal preferences for one health state relative to alternatives under uncertainty and is based on expected utility theory. Respondents are offered a choice between two alternatives, certain and gamble, which are presented with a decision tree.[30] To determine utility of certain health state i, an individual is asked to choose between this less desirable but certain chronic health state and a gamble offering to have an improved state of health for additional t years with probability p or immediate death with probability $(1 - p)$. Standard gamble assigns values of utilities for health states on a cardinal scale from 0 to 1 where perfect health has utility of 1 and death has utility of 0.

Use of the standard gamble approach is possible for determining preference values of health state i when one outcome of the gamble alternative is preferred to that certain state i and another one is less preferred to it; that is, the health state being valued must be intermediate between the two gamble outcomes in terms of preference.[35] An example of the standard gamble approach for measuring the utility of dialysis for patients with kidney failure, which in this case is assumed to be health state, i (Figure 3-2).

The subject is presented with two choices. Choice 1 is to gamble on a kidney transplant that has the possibility of two outcomes: A patient either returns to a

Figure 3-2 Standard Gamble Approach for Measuring Utility of Kidney Transplant versus Dialysis

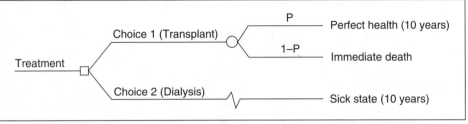

Source: Reprinted from Torrance GW. Measurement of Health State Utilities for Economic Appraisal. *J Health Econ,* 5(1):1–30. Figure 3, page 20, 1986. With permission from Elsevier.

desirable outcome, which is perfect health with probability p, or immediate death with probability $1 - p$. Choice 2 guarantees certain outcomes of the patient's health state for a certain number of years (or life) when the patient stays on dialysis. The interviewer varies probability p and asks the subject to select probability p^*, where the subject feels *indifferent* between the two choices. This indifference probability, p^*, is the utility value for the health state i according to the axioms of von Neumann-Morgenstern utility theory. For example, if a patient feels indifference between choice 1 and choice 2 when p^* is 0.9, then this patient is willing to accept a 10 percent risk of death to avoid the health state i $(1 - 0.9 = 0.1$ or 10 percent). Thus, utility of health state i (e.g., dialysis) is 0.9.

The advantage of the discussed approach is that in the standard gamble technique, an individual is faced with choices involving three health states (e.g., dialysis, death, perfect health) on an interval scale, what directly produces utilities with interval scaling properties. Standard gamble is considered a conservative utility measurement approach because the preference for the gain is much lower than the desire to avoid the loss when individuals are asked to choose between a gain and a loss of similar magnitude.[33] Individuals almost always prefer to stay at lower health state (e.g., dialysis) rather than bear substantial risk of death. This results in relatively high utility values stated by individuals in this approach.

Time Trade-Off Method

The **time trade-off method** (TTO) is another approach derived from expected utility theory for determining utility of health states, which constitutes comparisons between living longer at less-than-perfect health state versus having a specified shorter but healthy life.[37] TTO is an implicit approach, where preference values are derived implicitly from responses of individuals to decision situations.[35]

The TTO method is more facile for subjects than the standard gamble. This approach is not based on axioms of von Neumann-Morgenstern expected utility theory, but consistent with the axioms under strict assumptions. This approach offers health-time choices under certainty; an individual is presented with a certain choice that does not involve probability and risk. As a result, the preference estimated using the TTO method is considered a value score.[30] In general, the value score is lower than the utility score obtained from standard gamble for the same health state.[32]

The TTO approach for chronic health state preferred to death is shown in Figure 3-3. The subject is presented with two choices: 1 and 2. Choice 1 is a state in which an individual lives in perfect health for time (x), followed by death. Choice 2 is a state in which an individual lives in health state i for a certain time (t) followed by death (length of health state is life expectancy of the patient with health state i). The interviewer varies time in perfect health (x) to find the time (x^*, not shown in the figure), where the subject feels indifferent between choices 1 and 2. The subject is asked how many years of life he or she would be willing to give up to be in the perfect health state compared with the health state i.

The utility for the health state i is measured by the amount of time the subject is willing to give up to return to perfect health. Thus, the utility for health state i can be calculated by dividing x^* by t in Figure 3-3, and is represented as h.

Figure 3-3 Conceptual Illustration of the Time Trade-Off Method

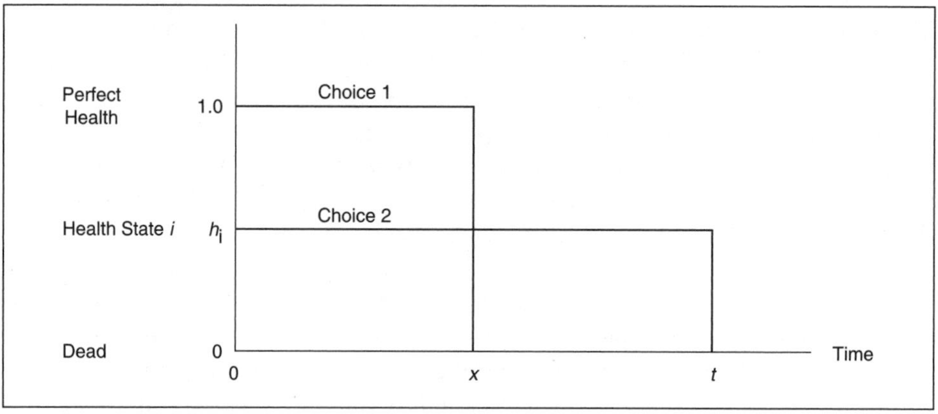

Source: Reprinted from Torrance GW. Measurement of Health State Utilities for Economic Appraisal. J Health Econ; 5(1):1–30. Figure 6, page 23, 1986. With permission from Elsevier.

Rating Scale Technique

Another direct measure of determining health utilities is the **rating scale technique**, which is sometimes referred to as a "feeling thermometer."[30] In this approach, health states are measured on the linear rating scale between anchors of 1 representing perfect health and 0 representing death. The interviewer instructs the individual to place the health states on the scale such that the intervals between their placements reflect the differences a person perceives between the health states and the relative desirability among levels.[30, 33] Like TTO, the rating scale does not involve uncertain outcomes, so the preference score generated is considered a value score.[38] Although the value obtained from this method is not a utility value, this method has been used as a warm-up method to the standard gamble or TTO methods. This method is useful for ordering outcomes by preference. The subject is asked to place the health state *i* in between death and perfect health state in Figure 3-4.

Figure 3-4 Graphical Illustration of a Health Utility Rating Scale

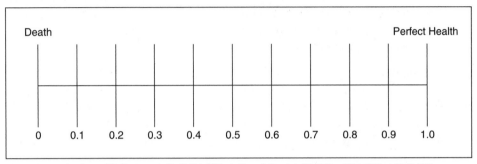

Source: Information from Torrance GW. Measurement of Health State Utilities for Economic Appraisal. *J Health Econ;* 5(1):1–30. Pages 18–20, 1986. With permission from Elsevier.

If there are several health outcomes to be ranked from most to least preferred, the outcomes that are almost equally desirable should be placed close to each other, whereas outcomes different in desirability should be placed far apart. When making a decision, an individual is asked to concentrate on the interval between health states rather than on scores in order to present the interval scale of preferences.[31]

Generic Instruments Used to Measure Utilities

Utility values also can be obtained by using one of the prescored multiattribute health status classification systems such as the European Quality of Life Index, Health Utility Index, Quality of Well-Being Scale, SF-6D, and others.

European Quality of Life Index

The **European Quality of Life Index** instrument, a multidimensional nondisease specific measure of health-related quality of life, presents a system for describing health status from Western Europe, which is capable of representing health status as a single index value.[39] A self-administered questionnaire contains questions attributable to five dimensions (mobility, self-care, usual activity, pain/discomfort, anxiety/depression) with each dimension having three levels of severity (no problem, some problems, major problems).[39, 40, 41]

The original EuroQol instrument contains six different dimensions: mobility, self-care, chief activity, social ability, pain/discomfort, and anxiety/depression, each with two or three levels. In the current version of the EQ-5D, chief activity and social ability were combined into the usual activity dimension.[39] Each patient is asked to report his or her health state in five dimensions, selecting only one level of severity for each dimension. Then a reported EQ-5D health state is converted to a score using the tables presenting values for each of 243 possible health states. Also included are death and unconsciousness or using the regression weights of the three levels of severity for each of the dimensions depending on which level for each dimension a person selects. Valuation of health states scores in EQ-5D are generated by TTO method, which is known to perform better than other methods in terms of internal consistency, reliability of the answers given by respondents, and sensitivity of valuations to parameters known to influence them.[42]

Health Utilities Index

The **Health Utilities Index** (HUI) is another generic approach used to measure health status and assess HR-QOL.[32] Because health status is a multidimensional concept, the HUI system uses a multiattribute approach in which a number of aspects of health status are specified using a comprehensive classification system. The HUI consists of two complementary components: a multiattribute health status classification system used to describe health status and a multiattribute utility function used to value health status as measured within the corresponding multiattribute health status classification system.

There are three HUI systems: HUI Mark I, HUI Mark II, and HUI Mark III. Each system has a health status classification system consisting of multiple levels of functioning across the attributes constituting a health state and one or more scoring formula. To use any of the systems, researchers must describe the health states of subjects based on HUI classifications and calculate the score using the corresponding formula. All scores are preference based (i.e., derived from the preferences of the general population), interval-scaled, and on the 0 (dead) to 1 (perfect health) scale.[31, 38]

HUI Mark I system was developed by Torrance and colleagues, is an extension of the multiattribute framework created to evaluate outcomes for very low birth weight infants. The system consisted of four attributes (physical function, role function, social-emotional function, and health problems) with four to eight levels of function for each and described 960 unique health states.[38] Preference scores were measured using the visual analogue and TTO technique.[33]

HUI Mark II, based on the HUI Mark I system, is a seven-attribute system (sensation, mobility, emotion, cognition, self-care, pain, and fertility) with each attribute consisting of four or five levels of specified impairment from no impairment to full impairment.[31, 38] This was initially a tool to assess health status in survivors of childhood cancer. Preferences for the scoring function were measured using both a visual analogue technique and a standard gamble instrument.[31]

Subsequently, the Mark II system was adapted for use in population health surveys and became the Mark III system.[38] In the new version, fertility was dropped; the sensory attribute was expanded to include vision, hearing, and speech; and other changes were made to increase the structural independence of the attributes, resulting in a total of eight attributes (vision, hearing speech, ambulation, dexterity, emotion, cognition, and pain). Preferences were measured using both a visual analogue and a standard gamble approach.

Quality of Well-Being Scale

The Quality of Well-Being (QWB) Scale summarizes current well-being and prognosis and is intended to be used both as a measure of needs for care and an outcomes measure for health program evaluation.[43] QWB consists of two sections:

1. Descriptions of functional states in the areas of mobility with three levels, physical activity with three levels, and social activity with five levels
2. A list of symptoms and problem complexes.[44]

The 21 complexes of symptoms and problems are intended to represent all possible symptomatic complaints that might inhibit function. If patients have several problems or symptoms, they are classified based on the symptom or problem that they find to be the most undesirable. Observable respondents' health states are placed on a scale between 0.0 (death) and 1.0 (full health) using preference weights of QWB classification categories obtained from a random sample of the general public.[33] QWB is available in two versions (i.e., interviewer or self-administered), but the interviewer-administered instrument is recommended because the self-administered questionnaire has resulted in considerable misclassification.

SF-6D

The **SF-6D**, a health state preference measure, was developed to incorporate preferences into its scoring algorithm.[45, 46] The SF-6D is based on six dimensions (physical functioning, role limitations, social functioning, pain, mental health, and vitality) of the Short Form 36 (SF-36), with each dimension having two to six levels, defining a total of 18,000 different health states. A total of 249 health states were valued by the U.K. general population using the standard gamble method; multiple regression models were estimated to predict health-state values for all 18,000 states defined by the SF-6D health-state classification.[45] SF-6D is an alternative to existing preference-based measures of health. Although some of its estimates have been inconsistent and the value of the poorest health states have been overestimated, SF-6D is more descriptive and therefore has a greater degree of sensitivity than prior instruments.[45]

Judgment or Literature

Utility values can also be estimated using judgment or obtained from the literature.[35] Judgment, the simplest method of obtaining health state utility, is usually made by the researcher, by physicians, or other experts. When using judgment, it is important to perform extensive sensitivity analysis to check robustness of analysis results. Utility values may also sometimes be obtained from the literature—though if doing so, it is important that the subjects, health states, and measurements used in these published studies are comparable to the population of interest and that the measurement instrument is both valid and reliable.

Conclusion

QOL and utilities are outcomes that are commonly incorporated into economic evaluations. The last 20 years have led to major advances in the methodology for measuring QOL, but much work still needs to be done. There is still debate over how it is defined, how it should be measured, and whether it is a concept that is applicable to certain populations (such as the elderly, in particular).[47, 48] The concept of health utility is particularly important to economic evaluation, because utility weighting is used to calculate QALYS—a common outcome measure in cost-effectiveness and cost-utility analyses. A variety of methods are used to measure health utilities, including the standard gamble, time trade-off, and rating scale techniques. Standardized instruments that yield utility values are also available.

Case Study

Patients with inflammatory bowel disease (IBD) may suffer from a variety of symptoms. In addition to the physiological symptoms associated with the disease, patients may be affected in other ways that affect the quality of their life. How might this disease affect a patient's mental outlook, their social relationships, the quality of their sleep, and their ability to perform at work? Each of these dimensions reflects the possible impact of this disease on a patient's life. Furthermore, if a patient has other chronic conditions, such as asthma, heart disease, diabetes, or arthritis, how might these additional conditions add to the burden? A study was undertaken to evaluate the impact of IBD and other chronic conditions on the QOL of patients with IBD. In order to gain a comprehensive picture of how patients are impacted, both a disease-specific and a generic health-assessment instrument were chosen. For the disease-specific measure, patients completed an instrument called the Inflammatory Bowel Disease Questionnaire (IBDQ), which provided detailed information about the severity of their bowel symptoms. For the global assessment instrument, patients completed the SF-36 questionnaire; this instrument provides eight scale scores on various dimensions of physical, mental and role functioning and two component summary scores. Research participants also filled out the Pittsburgh Sleep Quality Index (PSQI), the Work Productivity Assessment (WPA), and a questionnaire about any other physical or mental condition by which they are affected.

Study/Discussion Questions

1. What can the results of this study tell us about the burden of disease on patients with IBD?
2. Which dimensions of well-being and functioning are affected the most?
3. What is the relationship between bowel symptom severity, physical functioning, mental functioning, sleep quality, and work productivity?
4. How can the results of this study guide physicians in their treatment of patients with IBD?
5. How can the results of this study help to inform policy makers about the needs and concerns of patients with IBD?

Suggested Readings/Web Sites

Bootman JL, Townsend RJ, McGhan WF (eds). *Principles of Pharmacoeconomics*. 3rd ed. St. Louis, MO: Harvey Whitney Books Company; 2004.

Bowling A. *Measuring Disease: A Review of Disease-Specific Quality of Life Measurement Scales*. 2nd ed. Philadelphia: Open University Press; 2001.

CDC National Center for Chronic Disease Prevention and Health Promotion. "Health-Related Quality of Life." Available at: www.cdc.gov/hrqol.

Center for Health Evidence. Available at: www.cche.net/usersguides/life.asp.

Cramer JA, Spilker B. *Quality of Life and Pharmacoeconomic: An Introduction*. Philadelphia: Lippincott-Raven; 1998.

Euro-QOL. Available at: www.euroqol.org.

Fairclough DL. *Design and Analysis of Quality of Life Studies in Clinical Trials*. Boca Raton, FL: Chapman & Hall/CRC; 2002.

Fayers PM, Machin D. *Quality of Life: Assessment, Analysis, and Interpretation*. Chichester, NJ: John Wiley & Sons; 2000.

Health and Quality of Life Outcomes. Available at: www.hqlo.com.

King CR, Hinds PS (eds). *Quality of Life: From Nursing and Patient Perspectives*. 2nd ed. Sudbury, MA: Jones and Bartlett Publishers; 2003.

Mapi Research Institute. "Building the Science of Quality of Life." Available at: www.mapi-research.fr.index/htm.

Medical Outcomes Trust. Available at: www.outcomes-trust.org.

Muennig P. *Designing and Conducting Cost-Effectiveness Analyses in Medicine and Health Care*. San Francisco: Jossey-Bass; 2002.

O'Connor R. *Measuring Quality of Life in Health*. Elsevier/Churchhill Livingstone; 2004.

Patrick DL, Erickson P. *Health Status and Health Policy: Quality of Life in Health Care Evaluation and Resource Allocation*. New York: Oxford University Press; 1993.

Quality of Life Instruments Database. Available at: www.qolid.org.

Quality Metric. "Health Outcomes Solutions." Available at: www.qualitymetric.com.

Spilker B. *Quality of Life and Pharmacoeconomics in Clinical Trials*. 2nd ed. Philadelphia: Lippincott-Raven; 1996.

References

1. Kattan MW. Comparing treatment outcomes using utility assessment for health-related quality of life. *Oncology (Huntingt)*. 2003;17(12):1687–1693.

2. Roila F, Cortesi E. Quality of life as a primary end point in oncology. *Review Ann Oncol*. 2001;12 Suppl 3:S3–S6.

3. Wiklund I. Assessment of patient-reported outcomes in clinical trials: the example of health-related quality of life. [Review] *Fundam Clin Pharmacol*. 2004;18(3):351–363.

4. D'Amico D, Grazzi L, Usai S, Rigamonti A, Solari A, Bussone G. Measuring responses to therapy in headache patients: new and traditional end-points. *Neurol Sci*. 2004;25 Suppl 3:S108–S110.

5. Klassen AF, Miller A, Fine S. Health-related quality of life in children and adolescents who have a diagnosis of attention-deficit/hyperactivity disorder. *Pediatrics*. 2004;114(5):e541–e547.

6. Fairclough DL. Patient reported outcomes as endpoints in medical research. [Review] *Stat Methods Med Res*. 2004;13(2):115–138.

7. Cohen SB, Strand V, Aguilar D, Ofman JJ. Patient-versus physician-reported outcomes in rheumatoid arthritis patients treated with recombinant interleukin-1 receptor antagonist (anakinra) therapy. *Rheumatology* 2004;43(6):704–711.

8. Asadi-Lari M, Tamburini M, Gray D. Patients' needs, satisfaction, and health related quality of life: towards a comprehensive model. *Health Qual Life Outcomes*. 2004;2(1):32.

9. Fairclough DL. *Design and Analysis of Quality of Life Studies in Clinical Trials*. Boca Raton, FL: Chapman & Hall/CRC; 2002.

10. O'Connor R. *Measuring Quality of Life in Health*. St. Louis, MO: Elsevier/Churchhill Livingstone; 2004.

11. Spilker B. *Quality of Life and Pharmacoeconomics in Clinical Trials*. 2nd ed. Philadelphia: Lippincott-Raven; 1996.

12. King CR, Hinds PS (eds). *Quality of Life: From Nursing and Patient Perspectives.* 2nd ed. Sudbury, MA: Jones and Bartlett Publishers; 2003.

13. Bootman JL, Townsend RJ, McGhan WF (eds). *Principles of Pharmacoeconomics.* 3rd ed. Cincinnati: Harvey Whitney Books Company; 2004.

14. Tramarin A, Campostrini S, Postma MJ, Calleri G, Tolley K, Parise N et al. A multi-centre study of patient survival, disability, quality of life and cost of care: among patients with AIDS in northern Italy. *Pharmacoeconomics.* 2004;22(1):43–53.

15. Oliva J, Roa C, del Llano J. Indirect costs in ambulatory patients with HIV/AIDS in Spain: a pilot study. *Pharmacoeconomics.* 2003;21(15):1113–1121.

16. Turini M, Redaelli A, Gramegna P, Radice D. Quality of life and economic considera-tions in the management of prostate cancer. *Pharmacoeconomics.* 2003;21(8):527–541.

17. Prasad M, Rentz AM, Revicki DA. The impact of treatment for gastro-oesophageal reflux disease on health-related quality of life: a literature review. *Pharmacoeconomics.* 2003;21(11):769–790.

18. Mapes DL, Bragg-Gresham JL, Bommer J, Fukuhara S, McKevitt P, Wikstrom B et al. Health-related quality of life in the Dialysis Outcomes and Practice Patterns Study (DOPPS). *Am J Kidney Dis.* 2004;44(5 Suppl 3):54–60.

19. Ware JE, Snow KK, Kosinski M, Gandek B. SF-36® *Health Survey Manual and Interpretation Guide.* Boston: New England Medical Center, The Health Institute; 1993.

20. McHorney CA, Ware JE, Rogers W. et al. The Validity and Relative Precision of MOS Short- and Long-form Health Status Scales and Dartmouth COOP Charts: Results from the Medical Outcomes Study. *Med Care.* 1992;30(5):MS253–MS265.

21. Parkerson G. Duke Health Profile. Available at: healthmeasures.mc.duke.edu/images/DukeForm.pdf. Accessed May 30, 2005.

22. Bergner M, Bobbitt RA, Carter WB, et al. The Sickness Impact Profile: development and final revision of a health status measure. *Med Care.* 1981;19(8):787–805.

23. Jacobson AM, The DCCT Research Group: The diabetes quality of life measure. In *Handbook of Psychology and Diabetes.* Bradley C, (ed). Chur, Switzerland: Harwood Academic Publishers; 1994, 65–87.

24. Damiano AM, Steinberg EP, Cassard SD, Bass EB, Diener-West M, Legro MW et al. Comparison of generic versus disease-specific measures of functional impairment in patients with cataract. *Med Care.* 1995;33(4 Suppl):AS120–AS130.

25. Jolly M, Utset TO. Can disease specific measures for systemic lupus erythematosus predict patients health related quality of life? *Lupus.* 2004;13(12):924–926.

26. Ware JE, Jr., Kemp JP, Buchner DA, Singer AE, Nolop KB, Goss TF. The responsive-ness of disease-specific and generic health measures to changes in the severity of asthma among adults. *Qual Life Res.* 1998;7(3):235–244.

27. Engstrom CP, Persson LO, Larsson S, Sullivan M. Health-related quality of life in COPD: why both disease-specific and generic measures should be used. *Eur Respir J.* 2001;18(1):69–76.

28. Sprangers MA, Moinpour CM, Moynihan TJ, Patrick DL, Revicki DA. Clinical Significance Consensus Meeting Group. Assessing meaningful change in quality of life over time: a users' guide for clinicians. [Review] *Mayo Clin Proc.* 2002;77(6):561–571.

29. Symonds T, Berzon R, Marquis P, Rummans TA. Clinical Significance Consensus Meeting Group. The clinical significance of quality-of-life results: practical considerations for specific audiences. [Review] *Mayo Clin Proc.* 2002;77(6):572–583.

30. Haddix A. *Prevention Effectiveness.* Oxford: Oxford University Press; 2003.

31. Drummond M, O'Brien B, Stoddart G, Torrance G. *Methods for the Economic Evaluation of Health Care Programmes.* 2nd ed. New York: Oxford University Press; 1997.

32. Feeny D, Torrance GW, Furlong W. Health Utilities Index. *Quality of Life and Pharmacoeconomic in Clinical Trials.* Philadelphia: Lippincott-Raven; 1996.

33. Gold M, Siegel J, Russell L, Weinstein M. *Cost-effectiveness in Health and Medicine.* New York: Oxford University Press; 1996.

34. Sox H, Blatt M, Higgins M, Marlton K. *Medical Decision Making.* Boston: Butterworth-Heineman; 1988.

35. Torrance GW. Measurement of health state utilities for economic appraisal. *J Health Econ.* 1986;5(1):1–30.

36. Torrance GW. Preferences for health outcomes and cost-utility analysis. *Am J Manag Care.* 1997;3 Suppl:S80–20.

37. Torrance GW, Feeny D. Utilities and quality-adjusted life years. *Int J Technol Assess Health Care.* 1989;5(4):559–575.

38. Feeny D, Furlong W, Boyle M, Torrance GW. Multi-attribute health status classification systems. Health Utilities Index. *Pharmacoeconomics.* 1995;7(6):490–502.

39. Kind P. *The EuroQol Instrument: an index of health-related quality of life.* Philadelphia: Lippincott-Raven, 1996.

40. Brooks R. EuroQol Group. EuroQol: the current state of play. *Health Policy.* 1996;37(1):53–72.

41. Essink-Bot ML, Stouthard ME, Bonsel GJ. Generalizability of valuations on health states collected with the EuroQol-questionnaire. *Health Econ.* 1993;2(3):237–246.

42. Dolan P. Modelling valuations for health states: the effect of duration. *Health Policy.* 1996;38(3):189–203.

43. Wilkin D, Hallam L, Doggett M. *Measures of Need and Outcome for Primary Health Care.* New York: Oxford University Press; 1994.

44. Kaplan RM, Anderson JP. A general health policy model: update and applications. *Health Serv Res.* 1988;23(2):203–235.

45. Brazier J, Roberts J, Deverill M. The estimation of a preference-based measure of health from the SF-36. *J Health Econ.* 2002;21(2):271–292.

46. Brazier JE, Kolotkin RL, Crosby RD, Williams GR. Estimating a preference-based single index for the Impact of Weight on Quality of Life-Lite (IWQOL-Lite) instrument from the SF-6D. *Value Health.* 2004;7(4):490–498.

47. Hendry F, McVittie C. Is quality of life a healthy concept? Measuring and understanding life experiences of older people. *Qual Health Res.* 2004;14(7):961–975.

48. Holland R, Smith RD, Harvey I, Swift L, Lenaghan E. Assessing quality of life in the elderly: a direct comparison of the EQ-5D and AQoL. *Health Econ.* 2004;13(8):793–805.

Chapter 4

HEALTH-RELATED PRODUCTIVITY

Nikita Patel, PharmD
Jennifer H. Lofland, PharmD, MPH, PhD
Laura T. Pizzi, PharmD, MPH

Overview

Healthcare costs in the United States have risen dramatically. In response, healthcare purchasers have implemented various strategies aimed at cost containment, such as contracting with healthcare organizations, limiting an individual's choice of health plans, and cost-shifting. With limited resources available, society and healthcare policy makers must be able to determine the value of pharmaceuticals or healthcare interventions to both purchasers and consumers.

Typically, the estimation of healthcare costs is based on direct expenses related to medical care, such as the cost of medications, hospital stay, and physician visit. The total impact of direct and indirect costs on employers' balance sheets provides the true costs attributable to the health conditions of its employees. Hence, it is imperative to understand the relationship between employees' health and their ability to work. The morbidity and mortality of workers results in the utilization of resources in the form of replacement of workers—including new hires and temporary employees, training new employees, and the decreased efficiency of the new worker to complete the job—all leading to costs incurred by employers.[1, 2]

For a true representation of the economic evaluation of a disease state, it is essential to include both direct medical costs and the indirect costs resulting from the time lost from work, this encompasses both absence from work, and reduced performance while on the job. In doing so, one must be able to recognize and appraise the available surveys and instruments that capture lost productivity to confirm their applicability to specific work environments.

This chapter describes the current state of affairs of lost productivity measurement, details the techniques of valuing lost productivity, and describes available productivity instruments and datasets. In addition, the chapter addresses the hurdles that policy makers must overcome to incorporate productivity measurement and assessment into healthcare decision making.

■ Learning Objectives

1. To be familiar with the relevant terms that aid in understanding productivity
2. To recognize the significance of lost productivity due to health conditions
3. To recognize how lost productivity is a public health concern
4. To identify and comprehend the methods used to value lost productivity
5. To identify the advantages and limitations of available lost productivity measurement instruments
6. To recognize databases that capture lost productivity

■ Keywords

Absenteeism
Angina-Related Limitation Work Questionnaire
Auxiliary time
Direct costs
Friction cost approach
Friction period
Handle time
Health and Work Performance Questionnaire
Human capital approach
Indirect costs
Lost (indirect) productivity costs
Medical Expenditure Panel Survey
Midlife Developmental Inventory
Migraine Work and Productivity Loss Questionnaire
National Health Interview Survey
Osterhaus technique
Presenteeism
Stanford Presenteeism Scale
Value-based purchasing
Worker Productivity Index
Work Productivity and Activity Impairment

Introduction

Since the 1940s, large employers have been the principal purchasers of healthcare benefits in the United States.[3] One hundred and sixty-one million nonelderly Americans are members of an employer-sponsored health plan.[4] Healthcare costs have escalated dramatically with premiums rising 11.2 percent in 2004 as compared to 2003; this is indicative of a continued trend of double-digit premium increases.[5] For the same fiscal year, the inflation rate as well as growth in employee earnings lagged behind increases in premiums by 9 percent points—such economical disparities provide a clearer perspective about the gravity of phenomenal increases in premiums.[6]

U.S. employers lose billions of dollars in lost productivity per year due to painful conditions.[7] What is the significance of this data—and data pertaining to other health conditions—to U.S. employers? How does one attach a dollar value to decreased efficiency at work and days missed from work? What are the implications of these dollar values to employers and policy makers? This chapter attempts to address these questions in an effort to elucidate a complex and sometimes controversial topic that is, none the less, critically important. We will discuss the significance of lost productivity and its relevance to the field of public health, as well as measurement and valuation approaches. Finally, we will discuss the challenges in measuring health-related productivity and conveying its meaning to employers and healthcare policy makers.

Background

Typically, investigations aimed at quantifying the burden of illness incorporate **direct costs** such as medical claims and pharmacy claims data. However, the **indirect costs** resulting from days absent from work and on-the-job losses, are usually not included. When money is exchanged for a healthcare product or service, a direct cost is incurred. In contrast, with indirect costs, money is not actually exchanged for goods or services. Indirect costs, also known as **lost (indirect) productivity costs**, are defined as "the value of production loss to society due to illness, with respect to paid as well as unpaid labor."[8] Though complex, for certain diseases, such as migraine headaches, musculoskeletal pain, and seasonal and perennial allergic rhinitis, indirect costs account for a significant portion of the costs associated with the condition or disease.

The necessary components to determine indirect or lost productivity costs are **absenteeism** and **presenteeism**. While the former is defined as the number of days missed from the workplace or nonwork activities, presenteeism illustrates the extent to which an employee is functioning while working.[9, 10] Presenteeism refers to an individual who is present at work but because of health problems is unable to be 100 percent efficient. Examples of decreased efficiency may include time spent on the phone, inferior work output, decreased work output, and chronic poor health.[10] Many of the instruments available to measure lost productivity are based on subjective methods (such as a patient self-report) to estimate the absenteeism and presenteeism associated with a disease. Because the majority of these data are subjective, it is challenging for employers and others to understand the true indirect costs associated with lost productivity.

Significance of Productivity to U.S. Employers

The advent of the 2004 fiscal year yielded an average increase of 12 percent in employer health insurance premiums as compared to the previous year.[11] Escalating premiums are a threat to profit margins forcing employers to resort to cost sharing and issuing personal health plans to curb costs.[12, 13] Employer awareness of the complementary nature of worker health and lost productivity has mounted during the last few years.[14, 15] The upward trend of healthcare costs, surpassing annual increases in gross domestic product, has led to an employer movement to ensure value when purchasing health benefits.[16]

Value-based purchasing (VBP) is defined as "organized attempts by purchasers to ensure and improve the quality of health programs when negotiating costs with providers and insurers."[16] AlthoughVBP is not sought to improve work productivity per se, in theory, it will if the result is that quality health care is delivered to a firm's employees. More importantly, the VBP movement represents that employers are aware of the importance of a healthy workforce—and an interest in understanding the impact of health conditions on employees' workplace productivity.

Employers are beginning to recognize that higher profits are directly related to a healthy work force.[15] The morbidity and mortality experienced by workers has economic consequences to the employer: the replacement of workers, the hiring of temporary employees, the training of new employees, inadequate usage of expensive equipment, administrative expenses in the form of additional paperwork, overtime compensation to other employees, and reduced overall productivity of employees undertaking additional work (implying a decrease in profits).[17]

A 1998 benchmarking study of health and productivity management programs that were implemented at 43 U.S. companies demonstrated that the median annual cost of such programs amounted to $9992 per employee.[18] This included costs incurred due to group health, turnover of employees, unscheduled absences, nonoccupational disability, and worker's compensation. Managers who view these types of expenses as unrelated will be unaware of the lost productivity costs to the firm. Remarkably, the study suggested that a savings of $2562 per employee per year would be realized by uniting these components and achieving "best practice targets" for expenditures. Though employers understand the logical relationship between employee health and productivity, strong data confirming this belief is scarce.

Lost Productivity: A Public Health Concern

Public health practitioners as well as policy makers possess a common goal: to seek interventions that reduce a population's morbidity and mortality. Certain acute and chronic illnesses have pervasive effects on the workplace. Engaging in activities that prevent the illness itself or curb its symptoms is attractive for policy makers due to the incentive of decreased health care expenditures and work loss. Furthermore, such actions align with community preventive health initiatives of public health services.

One example of a community preventive health intervention that may significantly impact work productivity is influenza vaccination. Annual morbidity and mortality associated with influenza are in the range of 50 million illnesses and 47,200 deaths.[19] However, according to the Advisory Committee on Immunization Practices, populations that should be vaccinated are persons aged 65 years or older and under 5 years, and those who are at risk of contracting influenza as a complication of other conditions (such as immune compromised individuals).[20] As a consequence of these recommendations, only 16 percent of individuals between the ages of 18 to 49 years were vaccinated for influenza (CDC 2001 data).[21]

Several studies on the cost and benefits of vaccinating working adults have demonstrated that the number of work days lost due to each occurrence of influenza per person ranges from 0.79 to 3.4 while a simulation model estimate revealed that influenza vaccination would prevent 12.3 days missed from work per 100 persons vaccinated.[22, 23, 24] This translates into total net savings of approximately $14 per person. Some studies attribute a net cost range of $11 to $66 per vaccination to vaccinate a healthy working individual depending on the match between circulating strains of influenza in a population and those strains contained in the vaccine, while a randomized controlled trial demonstrated a net savings of $47 per person.[22,25] Two major conclusions can be drawn from these studies advocating the practice of preventive medicine in working age individuals:

1. Forgone productivity in the form of absenteeism is a direct consequence of influenza
2. The savings due to fewer missed work days is the basis for a possible business case advocating vaccination of young individuals against influenza

Ill employees are prone to calling in sick and their productivity can be decreased substantially while on the job. In 2002, U.S. employees lost almost 4000 hours of work (absenteeism and presenteeism) due to pain conditions such as headache, arthritis, back pain, and musculoskeletal pain, contributing to an economic burden of $61 billion.[7] Adequate evidence exists for migraines, allergic rhinitis, and depression as well; monthly cost per migraneur due to productivity loss is $112.99 (in USD, 1996), while in the case of allergic rhinitis, the choice of drug to treat the ailment itself demonstrated a 5 percent increase in work productivity.[26] These data support the idea that public health and productivity go hand in hand.

▮ Theoretical Approaches for Assigning a Value to Productivity

How does one derive a dollar figure for lost workplace productivity? Two schools of thought exist for monetizing or placing a dollar value on lost productivity: the **human capital approach** (HCA) and the **friction cost approach** (FCA).[27, 28]

Introduced in the 1960s, the HCA appears to be the more frequently adopted method based on current literature. Simplicity and ease of use are the HCA's most notable characteristics. It is a function of an individual's wage, with 1 hour of lost productivity equal to 1 hour of pay.[26,28] In addition, one of the basic assumptions of the HCA method is that there is full use of labor or, in other words, no unemployment. Productivity losses are calculated from the beginning of the illness until the time of recovery or the end of the age of gainful employment.[27, 28]

Essentially, the HCA is used to estimate the *potential* loss from productivity, though the *actual* losses that the society or employer have suffered may be generally smaller in magnitude.[2] According to this method, the individual is thought to be a producer; as a result if one is unpaid, they are considered not producing and his work productivity is valued as $0.

From the employer's perspective, the HCA is a straightforward approach for the estimation of indirect costs. The HCA places a $0 value for those who are not paid to "work" such as homemakers and the elderly.[2] In such cases, this approach may not provide a true picture of one's actual productivity because wage may not be an appropriate measure of one's total lost productivity. The method undervalues the societal productivity of nonworking individuals—even though these people often perform important and valuable functions in society.

The second approach for valuing lost productivity is the FCA. The FCA is a relatively newer approach that was launched in 1992 by Koopsmanschap.[8] With the FCA, the **friction period** is the time required to replace a sick worker. The friction cost is defined as the cost of hiring, replacing, and training new employees, as per the Panel on Cost Effectiveness in Health and Medicine (discussed in

Chapter 2).[29] However, according to Koopsmanschap and van Ineveld, the friction costs should also include the productivity lost prior to absent workers being replaced and the decreased productivity output associated with these new employees. The foundation of the FCA lies in the assumption that, after a friction period, a currently unemployed individual will replace the absent worker provided that the level of unemployment is above the frictional unemployment level.

In the case of a long-term absence, assuming that sick individuals are always replaced by unemployed individuals may not be practical in the U.S. economy, where there is a relatively low rate of unemployment. The FCA takes the societal perspective because the additional societal costs (i.e., cost of hiring and replacing new employees) are included in the cost estimations and the original worker's absence is no longer valued once he or she has been replaced.[8] Koopmanschap and van Ineveld have suggested that (1) absences shorter than those that lead to worker replacement should be valued as only 80 percent of the production value lost in that period; and (2) one half of the absences that are less than one week do not have indirect costs, because this work may be cancelled or postponed.

With the existence of two varied approaches, there have been discussions concerning which is the most appropriate methodology to calculate productivity. To illustrate the differences between the HCA and FCA methods, consider a manuscript by Lofland and associates.[30] A secondary, retrospective analysis was conducted to examine the differences in the estimations of lost productivity between the HCA and FCA. The original study was conducted in individuals with migraine headache who had recently begun using a migraine-specific medication. Productivity information was collected via self-administered surveys that were collected at baseline, 3 months, and 6 months after the initiation of the migraine-specific therapy. Six months after commencing the treatment regimen, results demonstrated totals amounting to $117,905 and a range of $28,329 to $117,905 in productivity losses using the HCA and the FCA, respectively.

The study showed that depending on the assumptions used, the FCA can yield lost productivity estimates that vary greatly, from as little as 24 percent up to 100 percent of the HCA estimate. This wide variation illustrates that some of the assumptions and suggestions posed by Koopmanschap and van Ineveld in the FCA need to be examined further.

Chronic episodic diseases (e.g., migraine headache, asthma) may consist of frequent but relatively short periods (1–3 days) of lost productivity. Are these short absences simply additive so that the total lost productivity is simply the sum from each episode? Or is it that by having short absences repeatedly, the total lost productivity is greater than additive?

What if an employer feels that there is only lost productivity when a replacement or temporary employee has to be hired? The FCA states that lost productivity is confined to the period needed to replace a sick worker and that one half of absences of less than 1 week do not have a friction period.[24] Therefore, according to the FCA, if a replacement worker is not hired, then there is no productivity loss. Research has shown findings contrary to this assumption of the FCA. If a person is unable to effectively perform work duties because of health condition, he or she may actually have lost productivity (i.e., presenteeism), regardless of whether a replacement employee is hired.

Evidently, the method of placing a dollar value on lost productivity has not received unanimous acceptance by experts in the field. Overall, the assumptions incorporated into the investigation, length of absence, simplicity of the preferred approach, and the nature of the disease state must be taken into consideration.

◼ Measurement Methods

We have discussed two possible methods by which to value or monetize lost productivity. However, if a researcher or an employer was interested in measuring an individual's lost productivity, how would they go about it? What items should be collected? Should absenteeism, presenteeism, or both be collected? If one uses a survey, how does the employer determine if it's appropriate and scientifically valid?

Lost productivity due to chronic conditions amounts to an estimated annual cost of $234 billion to the nation.[31] Although the breadth and depth of available productivity data is currently limited, it is important to realize that indirect costs associated with a disease can be significant. An avenue that one might explore to obtain data on workplace absenteeism is the human resources department within a firm. One needs to be aware that the archival data from a human resources department usually only documents long absences in a detailed fashion, does not provide information about the responsible disease state, and some sick workers may use vacation days if they have used up the allotted personal or sick days.[32]

Because these data may be unreliable, many studies use patient-reported measures of lost productivity.[33-44] Currently, the use of questionnaires to determine employee reported workplace productivity is an accepted method. An ideal instrument would capture both absenteeism and presenteeism. Additionally, an instrument that is both reliable and valid is considered to be ideal.[47] For a comparison of the currently available health-related work productivity instruments, refer to Table 4-1 on page 73. Some of the more commonly used instruments are highlighted below.

The **Work Productivity and Activity Impairment** (WPAI) questionnaire is available in several versions dealing with various conditions. It was also designed as a self-administered questionnaire to assess absenteeism and presenteeism within clinical trials. The WPAI is available in numerous languages.[33,34]

In comparison to the WPAI, the **Worker Productivity Index (WPI)** is unique because it incorporates objective measures in addition to subjective measures.[35] Although this is not the prototypical instrument for measuring lost productivity, it is a good example of objectively trying to capture rates of absenteeism.

The WPI was specifically designed to measure the lost productivity for a population of telephone customer service employees.[35] Through the use of a computer-based system, the total time an employee is working at a workstation is electronically monitored. Variables that were combined to create two productivity measures include handle time and auxiliary time. **Handle time** was defined as the sum of an employee's talk time, transfer or hold time, and the time for follow-up work for each answered call. **Auxiliary time** referred to the amount of time in which an employee is unavailable to receive telephone calls at the workstation. This objective information is used to determine the worker's absenteeism.

The subjective component of the WPI includes evaluating the accuracy of information and interpersonal skills provided by the customer service representatives themselves. The subjective component of the WPI is used to determine the presenteeism associated with the employee. These parameters are assessed by supervisors via the monitored telephone calls that employees have with customers.

The WPI may serve as a gold standard in the estimation of absenteeism data. Its use has been documented for tracking productivity loss in conditions such as mental health, respiratory diseases, digestive diseases, injuries, cancer, and hypertension, among others.[36] Significant expenses associated with a computer-based system may serve as an impediment to the extensive use of the WPI.

Health-related work productivity has been recognized as a global issue by the World Health Organization, which has participated in the development of an instrument with Harvard researchers. The **Health and Work Performance Questionnaire** (HPQ) is a self-administered survey that measures absenteeism, job-related accidents, and work performance, and was intended to compare individual-reported and employer-archived data using a global rating scale (from 1 to 10).[37] This instrument was tested in four professions: airline reservation agents, customer service representatives, automobile company executives, and railroad engineers, where it appears to be a valid.

The **Stanford Presenteeism Scale**, as the name suggests, assesses only presenteeism.[38] Overall loss in productivity will not be realized using this scale, however it might be helpful if the on-the-job losses are relevant.[38] It is a six-item questionnaire; however, its data cannot be converted to a monetary value.

If measuring the lost productivity of a particular disease or measuring the impact of a disease-specific health management program, disease-specific instruments are available. The **Angina-Related Limitation Work Questionnaire** (ALWQ), and **Migraine Work and Productivity Loss Questionnaire** (MWPLQ) measure absenteeism and presenteeism specifically for angina and migraine, respectively.[39,40,41] The **Osterhaus technique** is another method developed to measure productivity loss associated with an illness. This method includes a self-administered questionnaire for individuals suffering from migraine, which captures both absenteeism and presenteeism and allows for translation of productivity losses to a dollar value.[42]

Existing Sources of Productivity Data

What if you are interested in learning about the productivity lost among individuals with a particular disease such as diabetes mellitus? Due to limited resources you are not able to collect lost productivity data. Which source(s) would enable you to answer this question? One place to start is the currently available national databases that have collected productivity data.

Such databases enable healthcare purchasers, policy makers, and researchers to determine the productivity losses associated with specific diseases or occupations. Some of these databases are described below, with a more comprehensive list in Table 4-2.[48]

Medical Expenditure Panel Survey

The **Medical Expenditure Panel Survey** (MEPS) is a national questionnaire that collects data on the types, frequency, and costs of specific healthcare services that individuals in the United States utilize.[49] Within the household component survey of the MEPS, a respondent's workplace and nonworkplace absenteeism are captured. The MEPS includes the number of hours a respondent works per week as well as a respondent's hourly wage and occupation.

For workplace absenteeism, the respondent is asked the number of workdays missed in which he or she stayed in bed at least half of the day. Similarly for nonworkplace absenteeism, participants are asked the number of additional days in which they spent at least half a day in bed because of physical illness, injury, or a mental or emotional problem.

Midlife Developmental Inventory

The **Midlife Developmental Inventory** (MIDI) is an instrument developed as part of the National Survey of Midlife Development in the United States (MIDUS).[50] The MIDUS, as part of a collaborative project, was administered to a nationally representative sample of approximately 7200 noninstitutionalized, English-speaking adults to examine the patterns, predictors, and consequences of midlife development. All respondents were between 25 and 74 years of age.

Table 4-1 Selected Instruments to Measure Productivity

Instrument	Year Published	Productivity Metrics	Direct Monetary Conversion	Number of Questions	Administration	Disease States in Which Tested
Angina-Related Limitation Work Questionnaire (ALWQ)[39]	1998	Absenteeism Presenteeism	No	17 items	Paper Self-Administered	Angina
Endicott Work Productivity Scale (EWPS)[43]	1997	Absenteeism Presenteeism	No	25 items	Paper Self-Administered	Depression
Health and Labor Questionnaire (HLQ)[44]	1995	Absenteeism Presenteeism	Yes	4 modules	Paper Self-Administered	Migraine, bladder electrostimulation, knee surgery, hip prosthesis
Health and Work Questionnaire (HWQ)[45]	2001	Unable to determine with limited data	Unable to determind	27 items	Paper Self-Administered	Smokers
Health and Work Performance Questionnaire[37]	2002	Absenteeism	Yes		Self-Administered	Does not focus on disease states
Migraine Work and Productivity Loss Questionnaire (MWPLQ)[40, 41]	1999	Absenteeism Presenteeism	Yes	23 items	Paper Self-Administered	Migraine
Osterhaus Technique[42]	1992	Absenteeism Presenteeism	Yes	12 items	Paper Self-Administered	Migraine
Stanford Presenteeism Scale (SPS)[38]	2002	Presenteeism	No	6 items	Paper Self-Administered	Unable to determine due to limited data
Work Limitations Questionnaire (WLQ)[46]	2001	Presenteeism	No	25 items	Paper Self-Administered	Asthma, headache, depression, epilepsy, gastrointestinal disease, psychiatric disorders, osteoarthritis, rheumatoid arthritis
Work Productivity and Activity Impairment (WPAI) Questionnaire[33, 34]	1993	Absenteeism Presenteeism	Yes	6 items	Paper Self- & Interview Administered	Several
Worker Productivity Index (WPI)[36]	1999	Absenteeism Presenteeism	Yes		Computer-based learning	Mental health, respiratory, digestive, injury, musculoskeletal, DM, hypertension, cancer

Sources: [39]Lerner, et al., 1998; [43]Endicott and Nee, 1997; [44]Van Roijen, et al., 1996; [45]Shikiar, et al., 2001; [37]Kessler, et al., 2003; [40, 41]Lerner, et al. 1999 and Davies, et al., 1999; [42]Osterhaus, et al., 1992; [41]Davies, et al., 1999; [46]Lerner, et al., 2001; [33, 34]Reilly, et al., 1993 and Reilly Associates, 2004; [36]Burton, et al., 1998.

The MIDI captures workplace and nonworkplace absenteeism collectively. The respondent is asked the number of days, in the past 30, that he or she was "totally unable" to go to work *or* perform normal household activities due to their physical or mental health. In addition, the survey asks the respondent the number of hours worked per week, work status (e.g., full-time, part-time, or not working), and annual personal earnings.

National Health Interview Survey

The National Health Interview Survey (NHIS) is a health questionnaire that has been conducted annually by the National Center for Health Statistics (NCHS) and the CDC since 1957. It captures information on the health of the civilian, noninstitutionalized, household population within the United States.[52] The NHIS includes the number of hours a respondent works per week, a respondent's occupation, and a respondent's family income.

For workplace absenteeism, the respondent is asked the number of the days or half days missed from work because of illness or injury during the past 2 weeks. Of those workdays missed the respondent is to note the number in which he or she stayed in bed for more than half of the day. For nonworkplace absenteeism, participants are asked the number of days during the past 2 weeks that they stayed or were kept in bed more than half of the day because of illness or injury.

Challenges Associated with Productivity Measurement

The field of lost productivity has matured immensely over the last decade. New tools were developed to measure presenteeism and absenteeism, allow for the monetization of productivity data, as well as the determination of the relationship between specific health conditions and productivity. Such efforts are the driving forces for continued progress.

One of the greatest challenges today is obtaining an accurate estimate of presenteeism. On-the-job work loss is a significant component for true productivity estimates, yet the majority of existing instruments rely upon subjective data to represent an individual's presenteeism—and existing databases do not capture it. Presenteeism measurement becomes particularly daunting when white-collar occupations, sometimes referred to as "knowledge workers" are considered. In contrast, measurement for manufacturing jobs may be relatively easy because many of these occupations are associated with a physical and tangible activity (e.g., number of bottles capped, cars produced) in a given period of time.

Today's job market is largely hiring individuals responsible for the cognitive tasks as opposed to process-driven tasks (e.g., an assembly line). Alternative tools ought to be developed to account for executives, managers, and professionals who are not working to their full capacity due to an illness or medical condition.

Furthermore, because few of the existing instruments are suitable for direct translation to a monetary figure, their usefulness may be limited. This is particularly true for policy makers, where assigning a monetary value to productivity losses and gains assists in prioritizing the urgency of medical interventions as well as estimating the true costs of treatments.

Finally, instruments pertaining to specific disease states (e.g., MPWLQ) and/or occupations (e.g., WPI) are critical to capture and compare the causal relationship between productivity and diseases. However, their applicability is limited and cannot measure the productivity of a population suffering from more than one disease state. This gap in productivity assessment renders the development of a generic instrument competent in providing accurate information across all disease states and professions a high priority.

Summary and Conclusions

In this chapter, we have helped the reader become familiar with the relevant terms in the field as well as recognize the significance of productivity due to health problems and how it is a public health concern. We have identified the current methods for valuing productivity, presented the various instruments available to capture lost productivity, and highlighted some databases that are used to collect productivity data.

The overarching rationale for persistent growth in the field of productivity measurement is incorporation of such findings into cost-effectiveness and cost-benefit analyses facilitating better-informed decisions regarding the value of medications and disease management programs for the payers as well as patients.

Case Study

Migraine headaches have been associated with significant medical costs to the healthcare system, as well as pain and suffering by patients, and loss in productivity for employers. For the patient, migraine headaches result in debilitation during a migraine attack as well as impairment in physical, social, and mental health between attacks. In the United States alone, there are over 9 million patient visits a year to internal medicine and family practice physicians for migraine treatment. As a result, the economic burden of migraine is significant, both in terms of the direct costs for medical care as well as the indirect costs associated with patients' lost productivity at work. In 1992, researchers estimated that U.S. employers may lose up to $17 billion a year because of decreased productivity due to migraine and that patients spent 3 million days a month bedridden during migraine attacks.

Table 4-2 National Databases that include Productivity Data

Name of Database	Productivity Metrics Suitable for Translation into a Monetary Figure	Organization	Web Site	Public Access	Access Fee	Key Features
Behavior Risk Factor Surveillance System (BRFSS)[52]	• Workplace absenteeism • Nonworkplace absenteeism	Centers for Disease Control	www.cdc.gov/brfss /questionnaires/pdf-ques/ 2004brfss.pdf	Yes, via Internet	No	• Determines prevalence of risk Factors • A monthly telephone survey is administered via cluster sampling • Does not capture information on work status, therefore assumptions must be made
Community Tracking Study Household Survey (CTS)[53]	• Workplace absenteeism	Center for Studying Health System Change	www.hschange.org/ index.cgi?file=cts1	Yes, via Internet	No	• Data obtained from 60 randomly selected communities • Survey conducted every 2 years • General information regarding activities of daily living • Cannot estimate individual's lost productivity
Medical Expenditure Panel Survey (MEPS)[49]	• Workplace absenteeism • Nonworkplace absenteeism	Agency for Healthcare Research and Quality	www.meps.ahrq.gov	Yes, via Internet	No	• National questionnaire collecting data on types, frequency, and costs of specific healthcare services utilized • Household component captures number of work hours worked, respondent's hourly wage, and occupation
Midlife Developmental Inventory (MIDI)[50]	• Workplace absenteeism • Nonworkplace absenteeism	MacArthur Foundation Research Network on Successful Midlife Development	http://webapp.icpsr.umich. edu/cocoon/ICPSR-STUDY /03596.xml	Yes, via Internet	No (requires membership)	• All respondents were between 25 and 74 years old • Respondents are asked to report number of hours worked per week, work status, and annual earnings

National Health Interview Survey (NHIS)[51]	• Workplace absenteeism • Nonworkplace absenteeism	National Center for Health Statistics & Centers for Disease Control	www.cdc.gov/nchs/about/major/nhis/quest_data_related_doc.htm	Yes, via Internet	No	• Statistics are collected from an annual sample of 36,000–47,000 households • Number of hours worked, occupation, and family income are captured • Adjusted days missed for nonwork activities must be calculated
Current Population Survey (CPS)[54]	• Workplace absenteeism	Bureau of Census for the U.S. Bureau of Labor Statistics	www.bls.gov/cps/	Yes, via Internet	No	• Administered as a monthly questionnaire survey with a sample of 50,000 houses • Employment and unemployment data is collected • Nonworkplace absenteeism or presenteeism cannot be estimated from the information gathered

Sources: [52]CDC; [53]The Center for Health System Change; [49]Agency for Healthcare Research and Quality; [50]McArthur Foundation; [51]CDC; [54]U.S. Bureau of Labor Statistics

In addition, studies have shown that patients who have migraine headaches have a lower quality of life than do patients who have diabetes, hypertension, or depression. The effective treatment of migraine headaches has the potential to benefit not only patients but the health system as well. The serotonin (5HT1) receptor agonists, including but not limited to sumatriptan (Imitrex), have been shown to be a safe and effective treatments for acute migraine headache and associated symptoms. Sumatriptan was first introduced as a subcutaneous injection in 1993, followed by an oral formulation in 1995. In addition to providing relief during an acute migraine attack, the injection has been shown to improve health-related quality of life, decrease healthcare costs, and decrease workplace productivity lost.

As the medical director of a large regional health maintenance organization (HMO), you would like to conduct a prospective, observational study assessing the outcomes of migraineurs in your HMO who received their first prescription for sumatriptan. You would like to evaluate the migraineurs' use of healthcare services as well as their lost productivity. Consider how you would design this evaluation, and what tools or databases you would use to assess productivity.

Study/Discussion Questions

1. What are the two main components of lost productivity? Define each component.
2. For your investigation, would you like to collect one or both of the two components of lost productivity? Explain your reasoning.
3. You would like to determine the monetary value associated with the lost productivity of the migraineurs in the investigation. Which methodology—human capital approach or the friction cost approach—would you like to use and why?
4. What instrument do you propose to use in your study to collect the component(s) of productivity?
5. What are the advantages and disadvantages of your selected instrument?
6. What challenges do you anticipate with collecting productivity data in this investigation?
7. How should the presenteeism of knowledge or white-collar workers be measured or captured?
8. What monetary value should be placed on the absenteeism due to health conditions among homemakers? Zero dollars, the cost of a comparable domestic worker, salary commensurate on the individual's education, or a salary higher than the salary commensurate with the individual's education?

Suggested Readings/Web Sites

Johannesson M. The willingness to pay for health changes, the human capital cost approach and the external costs. *Health Policy*. 1996;36:231–244.

Koopmanschap MA, Rutten FF. A practical guide for calculating indirect costs of disease. *Pharmacoeconomics*. 1993;4(6):446–454.

Koopmanchap MA, Rutten FF, van Ineveld BM., et al. The friction cost method for measuring indirect costs of disease. *J Health Econ*. 1995;14(2):171–189.

Koopmanchap MA, van Ineveld BM. Towards a new approach for estimating indirect costs if disease. *Soc Sci Med*. 1992;34(9):1005–1010.

Lofland JH, Frick KD. Publicly available US national surveys that capture lost productivity. Expert Rev. *Pharmacoeconomics Outcomes Res*. 2002;2(5):485–494.

Lofland JH, Pizzi L, Frick KD. A review of health-related workplace productivity loss instruments. *Pharmacoeconomics*. 2004;22(3):165–184.

References

1. Koopsmanchap MA, Rutten FF, van Ineveld BM, et al. The friction cost method for measuring indirect costs of disease. *J Health Econ*. 1995;14(2):171–189.

2. Peeples PJ, Wertheimer AI, Mackowiak JI, McGhan WF. Controversies in measuring and valuing indirect costs of productivity forgone in a cost of illness evaluation. *J Res Pharmaceut Econ*. 1997;8(3):23–32.

3. Kuttner R. The American health care system. Employer-sponsored health coverage. *N Eng J Med*. 1999;340(3):248–252.

4. Fronstin P. Sources of health insurance and characteristics of the uninsured: analysis of the March 2003 Current Population Survey, December 2003, Issue Brief no. 264. Available at: www.ebri.org/ibex/ib264.htm. Accessed May 19, 2005.

5. Kaiser Family Foundation and Health Research and Educational Trust—Employer Health Benefits. 2004 Summary of findings. Available at: www.kff.org/insurance/7148/. Accessed September 9, 2004.

6. U.S. Department of Labor, Bureau of Labor Statistics. Consumer Price Index, April 2004. Available at: ftp.bls.gov/pub/news.release/History/cpi.05142004.news. Accessed November 2, 2004.

7. Stewart WF, Ricci JA, Chee E et al. Lost productive time and cost due to common pain conditions in the US workforce. *JAMA*. 2003;290(18):2443–2454.

8. Koopmanchap MA, van Ineveld BM. Towards a new approach for estimating indirect costs if disease. *Soc Sci Med*. 1992;34(9):1005–1010.

9. Burton W, Conti D. The real measure of productivity. *Bus Health*. 1999; 17(11):34–36.

10. Loeppke R, Hymel PA, Lofland JH et al. Health-related workplace productivity measurement: general and migraine specific recommendations from the ACOEM Expert Panel. *J Occup Environ Med*. 2003;45(4):349–359.

11. Strunk BC and Ginsburg PB. Tracking healthcare costs: trends turn downward in 2003. Available at: content.healthaffairs.org/cgi/reprint/hlthaff.w4.354v1? Accessed August 11, 2004.

12. Galvin R, Milstein A. Large employers' new strategies in health care. *N Eng J Med.* 2002;347(12):939–942.

13. Robinson JC. Renewed emphasis on consumer cost sharing in health insurance benefit design. *Health Aff (Millwood).* 2002;Suppl Web Exclusives:W139-54. Available at: content.healthaffairs.org/cgi/reprint/hlthaff.w2.139v1. Accessed October 30, 2004.

14. Brandt-Rauf P, Burton WN, McCunney RJ. Health, productivity and occupational medicine. *J Occup Environ Med.* 2001;43(1):1.

15. Berger ML, Howell R, Nicholson S, Sharda C. Investing in Healthy Human Capital. *J Occup Environ Med.* 2003;45(12):1213–1225.

16. Maio VM, Goldfarb NI, Carter C, Nash DB. Value-based purchasing: a review of literature. Report #63 The Commonwealth Fund. Available at: www.cmwf.org/usr_doc/maio_valuebased_636.pdf. Accessed August 24, 2004.

17. Berger ML, Murray JF, Xu J, Pauly M. Alternative Valuations of Work Loss and Productivity. *J Occup Environ Med.* 2001;43(1):18–24.

18. Goetzel RZ, Guindon AM, Turshen IJ, Ozminkowski RJ. Health and productivity management: establishing key performance measures, benchmarks, and best practices. *J of Occup Environ Med.* 2001;43(1):10–17.

19. Viboud C, Boelle P, Pakdaman K, Carrat F, Valleron AJ, Flahault A. Influenza epidemics in the United States, France, and Australia, 1972–1997. *Emerg Infect Dis.* 2004;10(4):32–39.

20. Centers for Disease Control and Prevention. Prevention and control of influenza. Recommendations of the advisory on immunization practices. Available at: www.cdc.gov/mmwr/preview/mmwrhtml/rr5208a1.htm. Accessed August 24, 2004.

21. Data from the National Center for Health Statistics—Vital Health and Health Statistics. Available at: www.cdc.gov/nchs/about/major/nhis/released200209/figure04_2.htm. Accessed August 27, 2004.

22. Bridges CB, Thompson WW, Meltzer MI, et al. Effectiveness and cost-benefit of influenza vaccination of healthy working adults: a randomized controlled trial. *JAMA.* 2000;284(13):1655–1663.

23. Kavet J. A perspective on the significance of pandemic influenza. *Am J Public Health.* 1977;67(11):1063–1070.

24. Nichol KL. Cost-benefit analysis of a strategy to vaccinate healthy working adults against influenza. *Arch Intern Med.* 2001;161(5):749–759.

25. Nichol KL, Lind A, Margolis KL, et al. The effectiveness of vaccination against influenza in healthy, working adults. *N Engl J Med.* 1995;333(14):889–893.

26. Burton WN, Morrison A, Wertheimer AI. Pharmaceuticals and worker productivity loss: a critical review of the literature. *J Occup Environ Med.* 2003;45(6):610–621.

27. Johannesson M. The willingness to pay for health changes, the human capital cost approach and the external costs. *Health Policy.* 1996;36(3):231–244.

28. Koopsmanschap MA, Rutten FF. A practical guide for calculating indirect costs of disease. *Pharmacoeconomics*. 1993;4(6):446–454.

29. Gold MR, Siegel JE, Russel LB, et al., eds. *Cost effectiveness in health and medicine*. New York: Oxford University Press; 1996.

30. Lofland JH, Locklear JC, Frick KD. Different approaches to valuing the lost productivity of patients with migraine. *Pharmacoeconomics*. 2001;19(9):917–925.

31. Hoffman C, Rice D, Sung HY. Persons with chronic conditions: their prevalence and costs. *JAMA*. 1996;276(18):1473–1479.

32. Greenberg PE, Birnbaum HG, Kessler RC, Morgan M, Stang P. Impact of illness and its treatment on workplace costs: regulatory and measurement issues. *J Occup Environ Med*. 2001;43(1):56–63.

33. Reilly MC, Zborzek AS, Dukes EM. The validity and reproducibility of a work productivity and activity impairment instrument. *Pharmacoeconomics*. 1993;4(5):353–365.

34. Reilly Associates Health Outcomes Research. Available at: www.reillyassociates.net. Accessed November 2, 2004

35. Burton WN, Conti DJ, Chen CY, Schultz AB, Edington DW. The role of health risk factors and disease on worker productivity. *J Occup Environ Med*. 1999;41(10):863–877.

36. Burton WN, Conti DJ. Use of an integrated system health data warehouse to measure the employer costs of five chronic disease states. *Dis Manag*. 1998;1:17–26.

37. Kessler RC, Barber C, Berglund P, et al. The World Health Organization Health and Work Performance Questionnaire. *J Occup Environ Med*. 2003;45(2):156–174.

38. Koopman C, Pelletier K, Murray JF, et al. Stanford presenteeism scale: health status and employee productivity. *J Occup Environ Med*. 2002;44(1):14–20.

39. Lerner DJ, Amick III BC, Malspeis S, Rogers WH, Gomes DR, Salem DN. The angina related limitations questionnaire. *Qual Life Res*. 1998;7(1):23–32.

40. Lerner D, Amick III BC, Malspeis S, et al. The migraine work and productivity loss questionnaire: Concepts and design. *Qual Life Res*. 1999;8(8):699–710.

41. Davies GM, Santanello N, Gerth W, Lerner D, Block GA. Validation of a migraine work and productivity loss questionnaire for use in migraine studies. *Cephalagia*. 1999;19(5):497–502.

42. Osterhaus JT, Gutterman DL, Plachetka JR. Healthcare resource and low labor costs of migraine headaches in the US. *Pharmacoeconomics*. 1992;2(2):67–76.

43. Endicott J, Nee J. Assessment measures for clinical studies: Endicott work productivity scale (EWPS): a new measure to assess treatment effects. *Psychopharmacol Bull*. 1997;33(1):13–16.

44. Van Roijen L, Essink-Bot ML, Koopmanchap MA, Bonsel G, Rutten FF. Labor and health status in economic evaluation of health care. The Health and Labor Questionnaire. *Int J Technol Assess Health Care*. 1996;12(3):405–415.

45. Shikiar R, Rentz AM, Halpern MT, Khan, ZM. The Health and Work Questionnaire (HWQ): An instrument for assessing workplace productivity in relation to worker health. *Value Health*. 2001;4(2):181.

46. Lerner D, Amick III BC, Rogers WH, Malspeis S, Bungay K, Cynn D. The Work Limitations Questionnaire. *Med Care*. 2001;39(1):72–85.

47. Lofland JH, Pizzi L, Frick KD. A review of health-related workplace productivity loss instruments. *Pharmacoeconomics*. 2004;22(3):165–184.

48. Lofland JH and Frick KD. Publicly available U.S. national surveys that capture lost productivity. Expert Rev. *Pharmacoeconomics Outcomes Res*. 2002;2(5):485–494.

49. Agency for Healthcare Research and Quality. Medical Expenditure Panel Survey. Available at: www.meps.ahrq.gov. Accessed August 24, 2004.

50. John D. and Catherine T. McArthur Foundation. Research Network on Successful Midlife Development (MIDMAC). National Survey of Midlife Development in the United States. Available at: midmac.med.harvard.edu/research.html. Accessed August 24, 2004.

51. Centers for Disease Control and Prevention. National Health Interview Survey. Available at: www.cdc.gov/nchs/about/major/nhis_dis/nhis_dis.htm. Accessed August 24, 2004.

52. Centers for Disease Control and Prevention. Behavior Risk Factor Surveillance System. Centers for Disease Control and Prevention. Available at: www.cdc.gov/brfss/. Accessed August 24, 2004.

53. The Center for Health System Change. Community Tracking Study Household Survey. Available at: www.hschange.org/index.cgi?file=cts1. Accessed November 2, 2004.

54. Bureau of Labor and Statistics. Current Population Survey. Bureau of Labor and Statistics. Available at: www.bls.gov/. Accessed August 24, 2004.

Chapter 5

ADJUSTMENTS WITHIN ECONOMIC EVALUATION

Craig S. Roberts, PharmD, MPA
Daniel E. Polsky, PhD

Overview

Economic evaluation of medical technologies requires that differences observed between treatments be attributable to the treatments and not caused by external factors. Quite often, data collected for economic evaluation are affected by patient or provider characteristics, local healthcare practice, or the effects of time on the perceived value of treatments. Therefore, in order to make fair comparisons between treatment options, adjustments may be required to costs and health outcomes in order to make appropriate conclusions about the value of healthcare interventions.

The use of observational data, or data collected from actual practice settings, often introduces substantial bias in the comparisons. Different treatments are frequently selected for different patients based on true or perceived differences in treatments. In the treatment selection process, patients with different characteristics receive different therapies and these patient characteristics may have a substantial influence on the observed outcomes. An economic evaluation must have a process to measure and correct for differences in patient characteristics in order to make valid comparisons.

In economic evaluation requiring long-term comparison of outcomes, changes in value over time can affect the comparison of outcomes between treatments. Outcomes that are observed immediately have greater value than outcomes that are observed far in the future. Correcting for time, or **discounting**, is an important adjustment that must be applied to studies that compare outcomes 1 year or greater into the future.

This chapter will describe efforts to improve the quality of economic evaluations by making adjustments to both outcomes and costs. It will detail why and when risk adjustment is important and the methods of applying it. It will also cover adjusting costs and outcomes for time using discounting.

Learning Objectives

1. To understand why adjustments to outcomes are often needed in economic evaluation
2. To describe common risk assessment tools for evaluating risk in patient populations
3. To describe different approaches to correct for differences in risk in economic evaluation
4. To identify when discounting must be applied to costs and outcomes in economic evaluation
5. To apply basic risk adjustment principles to a hypothetical economic evaluation

Keywords

Before-after design
Bias
Charlson Comorbidity Index
Comorbidities
Cross-sectional design
Difference-indifference design
Discounting
Discount rate
Elixhauser method
External validity
Inflation
Internal validity
Instrumental variable
Matched samples
Multivariate analysis
Patient risk
Propensity score
Randomization
Regression analysis
Risk
Risk adjustment

Risk factor
Selection bias
Validity

 Introduction

The purpose of economic evaluation of medical interventions is to aid decision makers in achieving an efficient use of healthcare resources at a community level by quantifying the trade-offs between changes in the resources devoted to health care and the resulting changes in health outcomes. For economic evaluations to achieve this purpose, it is necessary to adjust raw comparisons of outcome data collected from patients receiving different treatment options. Although it seems like a straightforward task, comparing data collected outside of a controlled environment frequently leads to misleading conclusions. Differences in provider perception, patient health, health system structure, and timing can all influence the outcomes we are trying to measure independent of the treatment itself. Economic evaluations that compare outcomes between treatments should reflect the effect of treatment on outcomes rather than the effect of other factors on outcomes. The primary objective of this chapter is to introduce adjustments in economic evaluation that lead to valid conclusions regarding the relationship between treatment and outcome.

Outcomes researchers measure the effects of medical interventions on the health and well-being of patients in nonexperimental and quasiexperimental studies. Observational datasets are frequently used for such research because they allow us to study the effects of treatments in a real-world setting. These datasets include billing systems used by managed care organizations or hospitals that track services delivered to patients or electronic medical record systems used to organize patient medical history in a physician practice. Although these datasets provide large sources of information on treatments and outcomes in true practice settings, the complexity of clinical practice can interfere with interpretation of observed data.

If we are not comparing two treatment groups that are alike in every way except for the treatment received, it is possible that the conclusions of the research will be misleading. To convincingly assign measured outcome differences to the effect of treatment rather that the effect of other factors is a great challenge in economic evaluation. The medical establishment has embraced randomized clinical trials because this study design has been shown to be effective in overcoming this challenge. Randomization reduces the likelihood that other factors cause differences between outcomes leaving one to conclude that the treatment itself is the cause of the different outcomes.

When randomized experimental designs are not possible, we must attempt to make conclusions about causality from observed relationships. However, an observed relationship does not imply causality. For example, no one believes that carrying an umbrella will make it more likely to rain. However, if we were to look out our window in the morning and count the number of people carrying umbrellas, and then later record the occurrence of rain, we would find that there is a relationship between carrying umbrellas and rain. Despite this observed relationship, we would not conclude that umbrellas caused the rain because of our understanding of how rain occurs and why people carry umbrellas.

Similarly, patients who have more severe illness are more likely to seek out the best physicians. Patients who have more severe illness are also likely to have poorer outcomes. Therefore, in research of observational data, it is common to observe a positive relationship between better physicians and worse outcomes. It would be a mistake to conclude that these physicians cause the worse outcomes, because it is more likely the severity of the patient that is driving the difference in outcome. Similarly, it would be a mistake to conclude that umbrellas cause rain. Because these issues are regularly faced when analyzing these data, the quality of economic evaluation is often dependent on making corrections for these differences so that accurate conclusions can be reached. This chapter will discuss adjustments that need to be made in economic evaluation to ensure the conclusions of economic studies are indeed correct.

Validity and Bias

Validity is the extent to which the results of a study correctly answer what the study was designed to answer. Validity can refer to **internal validity**, or the extent to which the study makes correct conclusions about the subjects in the study, or **external validity**, the extent to which the study results make correct inferences about the population as a whole. An example of poor internal validity is a study that compares outcomes between those who receive two different therapies in which those who receive one therapy were severely sick when they entered the study, while those who received the other therapy were only slightly sick. The treatments received by different groups cannot be compared, and the study cannot make conclusions about the differences. An example of poor external validity is using a study in an elderly population to make claims about a middle-aged population.

One of the most common limiting factors of internal validity is bias. **Bias** is a difference in observed outcomes between study groups that results from a systematic difference in factors not related to treatment. In observational studies, where treatment selection is typically determined by clinical judgment, perceptions of the strengths and weaknesses of treatments are the factors that determine which patients are in which treatment group. Therefore, one treatment may be systematically used in older patients, patients with or without a particular comorbid disease, or patients with more severe disease under study. This is the systematic nature of bias—the factors that led to the selection of one particular treatment over another may also be factors that have great influence over the outcomes measured in a study.

One common type of bias in studies results from comparing two groups of patients who have different risk of having a poor outcome independent of treatment. **Risk** is the likelihood a particular person will experience a particular outcome during a specific period of time. A **risk factor** is a preexisting condition that increases a person's risk for an outcome. Risk factors are highly dependent on the outcome of interest. Common risk factors for poor health outcomes include older age, presence of chronic diseases, and smoking. When comparing cohorts of patients with different proportions of risk factors, the analysis may be subject to **selection bias**. This is bias generated by the reason treatment was selected. However, there are well-established adjustment methods to address this bias. The most prominent, **risk adjustment**, reduces bias by adjusting for the differences in risk factors among groups of patients.

In long-term studies, such as long-term observational studies or models with long-term outcomes, a different type of bias can affect the comparison of outcomes between treatments. This bias involves time, where outcomes that are observed immediately have greater value than outcomes that are observed far in the future. Although this bias does not involve selection or risk, correcting for time is an important adjustment that must be applied to studies that compare outcomes 1 year or greater into the future. This adjustment, referred to as discounting, will be addressed near the end of the chapter.

Risk Adjustment

Introduction

To conduct a meaningful comparison of patient outcomes using observational data, adjustment for patient risk is necessary in order to address the threat selection bias poses to the internal validity of the study. **Patient risk** can be defined by the factors that patients bring to healthcare encounters that could affect their outcomes. These factors include age, medical history, social support, motivation, and the ability to comply with medical therapy. The purpose of adjustment is to take these factors into account to level the playing field when making comparisons. By adequately controlling for patients' risk factors, we can draw useful inferences from observed healthcare outcomes about treatment effectiveness, provider performance, or quality of care.

Making fair comparisons and conclusions begins with a carefully planned study design to minimize the dependence on accurate risk adjustment by minimizing risk differences between groups. This must be followed by a well-constructed risk adjustment model, in order to correct outcomes for differences in risk.

Study Design

The best way to approach risk adjustment in a study is to minimize the need for risk adjustment by careful design of the study. Although this will not correct every problem with selection, study design can help identify and compare treatment groups that are most likely to be similar. By designing a study with an understanding of bias, many of the problems faced in analysis of outcomes data can be minimized.

The optimal solution to correct for selection bias is to randomly select patients to receive one treatment or another. Through **randomization**, any patient entering a study is equally likely to receive one study treatment of interest. This prevents treatment selection based on demographic characteristics or differences in patient risk. As a result, differences in risk between groups occur at random. This results in study groups that are balanced, or equivalent in terms of the underlying risk factors for future outcomes. An important but not obvious benefit of randomization is that it corrects not only for known differences in risk, but also unknown or unmeasured differences. This method is routinely employed in clinical trials for new medications.

One option would be to use randomized trials for all outcomes-research evaluations. However, randomized trials cannot be run for all medical decisions due to financial limitations, practical limitations, or ethical considerations. Such trials are very expensive and take a very long time to design, implement, and analyze. Plus, in order to be efficient and focused, randomized trials tend to enroll an extremely specific and limited patient population, limiting the generalizability of these comparisons in the broader population. Thus, because of randomization and minimal selection bias, randomized trials tend to have excellent internal validity, but they also tend to have poor external validity because of the narrowly defined sample of patients they compare.

Observational studies in economic research are often retrospective analyses of preexisting datasets. Unlike randomized trials, these retrospective observational studies do not require collection of new data, so they are often faster to complete and less expensive. They may also reflect true clinical practice better than randomized trials, because the data is a snapshot of the type of care patients receive in a noncontrolled true-practice environment. In retrospective observational studies, however, randomization is impossible, because we are looking in the past at patients who have already received treatment(s). Therefore, a researcher must be aware of bias from the beginning of the analysis in order to collect the data, measure it, and correct for it before initiating comparisons between study groups.

One basic approach for reducing differences in patient risk through study design is establishing well-defined inclusion and exclusion criteria. These criteria limit the patients being studied to a more focused and similar population. Commonly criteria limit a study to patients in a certain age range, patients with or without particular medical conditions, or patients treated in a particular type of healthcare setting. This approach can correct for large problems, but has great drawbacks as a stand-alone, risk-adjustment measure. First, it limits the generalizability of the conclusion to the narrowly defined sample studied. Second, it may limit the sample size of analysis and power of the results. However, it is generally useful to limit the study to the condition you are trying to treat. For example, if using retrospectively collected data to compare two hypertension treatments and one of the treatments is also used for unrelated conditions, such as migraine headache or congestive heart failure, it may be useful to limit the sample to only patients with documented hypertension who do not have migraine or heart failure.

Other approaches to minimizing the effects of selection bias in observational studies are study designs such as **before-after design** and the **difference-indifference design**. The before-after design looks at patients over time and captures their outcomes before and after treatment. The effect of treatment is measured as the change in their outcomes before and after treatment. In a medical setting, those subjects observed before treatment are typically observed at the point where they may be sickest because it is that health decline that sent them to treatment. It is not necessarily the case that the before-after change in outcome is the result of treatment because health may have improved even if treatment was not delivered. The difference-in-difference design attempts to overcome this limitation by adding a comparison group that is also observed before and after. The change in outcomes of one treatment group is compared to change in the other treatment group. These two designs work best when the opportunity for treatment is unanticipated or independent of baseline risk factors.

The most common design in economic analysis is a **cross-sectional design**. The key to successful measurement with this design is that the risk factors—after adjustment—are equivalent between the comparison groups. Therefore, in the process of this type of study design, one should anticipate and prepare a plan for risk adjustment. The plan should describe what risk data will be collected, how differences in risk will be assessed, and what methods will be applied to correct for differences between patients. Substantial and significant unanticipated differences in risk may necessitate additional secondary post-hoc analyses not anticipated prior to analysis of data; however, most risk differences can be well corrected through knowledge of the disease area and familiarity with risk-adjustment methods. Every effort should be made to provide comparisons that are as balanced as possible between the patient groups that are being compared.

The process for addressing this bias involves assessment of risk factors likely to cause bias, measurement of risk factors in the study groups, and application of methods to adjust or control for the difference in underlying risk. Other risk-adjustment methods seek to simulate comparisons among patients that are most likely to be similar, mimicking the effect of randomization. These risk-adjustment methods will be described in the next section of the chapter.

Measuring Risk

Measurement of risk involves collecting data to identify risk factors in the study and classifying them in a manner that makes them useful. Risk factors are best collected in the period immediately preceding the receipt of treatment(s) of interest to a study. This allows for most accurate and up-to-date measurement of risk, without the possibility of inadvertently including risk factors that develop as a consequence of treatment. Collection of appropriate risk factors will allow for comparison of risk in different comparison groups in economic evaluation and will allow for consideration of these differences in risk adjustment.

Collection of risk factors begins with an understanding of the disease process and known factors that affect the outcome under study. Research of prior literature, consultation of experts, or personal experience may be required to understand the known or suspected factors that are likely to influence outcome. Demographic factors are often included in risk assessment as they are often indicative of differences in risk or risk factors. Age, for example, is both independently associated with greater risk of many poor outcomes, including excess cost and higher mortality, and is associated with many other conditions that are also predictive of poor outcomes. Measures of disease severity, prior medical history, and co-occurring chronic disease are also important risk factors for consideration.

Data pertaining to the severity of the specific disease under study are critical to understanding differences in risk between patient groups. Many health conditions have well-defined indicators of greater severity. In hypertension, baseline blood pressure is an important indicator of poor outcome. In diabetes, glycocylated hemoglobin, an indicator of long-term blood sugar control, is an important predictor of poor outcomes.

In addition, past medical history often predicts future medical events. Medical events that are important to the outcome of a study should be captured in a defined period prior to the study. For example, if the results of economic analysis are likely to be driven by differences in hospital care, hospital care prior to treatment is a factor that should be collected. Similarly, in a study of patients with acute exacerbations of chronic bronchitis (AECB), the number of past exacerbations is an important factor that is likely to predict differences in cost and outcomes in patients.

Diseases other than the disease under study, or **comorbidities**, must also be considered as indicators of risk. Co-existence of chronic disease is a strong risk factor for many poor health outcomes, including mortality, hospital length of stay, and cost. Comorbidity often also has an effect on the care of patients and selection of treatment. Acknowledgment and interest in the effects of comorbid disease on patient outcomes have led to the development of several scoring systems to classify and rank patients with different severity of illness. These scoring systems often consist of a combination of demographic factors, clinical measurements, and presence of comorbid diseases into a score that is positively correlated with the probability of the outcome. These scores are frequently used for risk assessment and adjustment. An overview of several common risk scoring systems developed to predict mortality following hospitalization are included in Table 5-1.

Table 5-1 Measures of Risk Due to Comorbid Disease

Index	Purpose	Components	Output
Kaplan and Feinstein (1974)[1]	Rate comorbidity status by severity of most severe chronic illness to predict poor outcomes	Includes 12 conditions each clinically defined and rated as mild, moderate, or severe	Mild, moderate, or severe comorbidity
Charlson comorbidity index (1987)[2]	A weighted index that predicts risk of mortality from comorbid disease in 1- and 10-year periods	Includes 17 clinically defined serious medical conditions weighted by severity	Summary score from 0 to 31
Charlson comorbidity index, Deyo (1992)[3]	Adaptation of Charlson comorbidity index for billing data, using billing codes to classify diseases	Includes 17 serious medical conditions as above, defined by specific ICD-9 codes	Summary score from 0 to 31
Charlson comorbidity index, Romano (1993)[5]	Adaptation of Charlson comorbidity index for billing data, using billing codes to classify diseases	Includes 17 serious medical conditions as above, defined by specific ICD-9 codes	Summary score from 0 to 31
Elixhauser (1998)[6]	Identifies most important comorbidities predictive of in-hospital mortality and resource use using billing data	Defines 30 medical conditions using ICD-9 coding for classification	Thirty individual risk factors

Sources: [1]Kaplan and Feinstein, 1974; [2]Charlson, et al., 1987; [3]Deyo, et al., 1992; [4]Romano, et al., 1993; [5]Elixhauser, et al., 1998.

One of the earliest measures of comorbidity severity was developed by Doctors Kaplan and Feinstein in an analysis of patients with diabetes.[1] They collected data on diabetic patients from a veteran's administration hospital database to examine factors that predicted 5-year mortality. A rating system was established to grade the severity of multiple conditions, classified as hypertension, cardiac, cerebral or psychiatric, respiratory, renal, hepatic, gastrointestinal, peripheral vascular, malignancy, locomotor impairment, alcoholism, and miscellaneous. Each of these conditions could be assigned one of three grades, with grade 3 representing a life-threatening level of severity, grade 2 as potentially life threatening, and grade 1 as less severe. An individual patient was assigned a grade based on the grade of their most severe comorbid condition, unless they had two or more grade 2 ailments, at which they were assigned a grade 3. A patient with no qualifying conditions was a grade 0. Five-year mortality was 7 percent, 28 percent, 42 percent, and 69 percent for grades 0, 1, 2, and 3, respectively, thus confirming the importance of comorbidity as a factor associated with survival. This pivotal study underscored the importance of accounting for differences in comorbid disease when analyzing mortality rates in populations.

Many years following the Kaplan and Feinstein method, one of the most widely adopted measures of comorbidity-associated risk, the **Charlson comorbidity index**, was developed.[2] This index was designed to provide a tool that could combine the effects of multiple comorbidities into a single score predictive of short- and long-term mortality for use in long-term studies. By identifying the key comorbid conditions a patient has, assigning a weight based on their predictive ability, and summing these scores, each patient in a study is associated with a single level of risk based on the effects of their overall chronic conditions. This score has been found to be predictive of mortality in several populations and has been widely adopted as a risk-assessment tool for a variety of populations.

One limitation to Charlson's original index is its reliance on clinically defined classifications of comorbidity. These definitions require thorough investigation into patient's healthcare records to identify comorbid disease. More recently, several investigators have adapted the comorbidity index so that the comorbidities can be identified using billing data.[3, 4, 5] These methods have defined the comorbidities used to calculate the index as specific International Classification of Disease (ICD-9) codes. This allows for use of these methods on large computerized databases. Although this method provides much less precision in identifying disease, the Romano and Deyo adaptations of the Charlson comorbidity index described have proven predictive of a variety of poor health outcomes in large database studies.

A more recent comorbidity classification method introduced by Elixhauser et al., was developed with current data and was created from the beginning to be a tool to classify comorbidities using administrative data to measure their impact on hospital charges, length of stay, and mortality.[6] Unlike the Charlson and Kaplan-Feinstein methods, the **Elixhauser method** is a system of classifying a list of billing codes into comorbidities that are predictive of poor outcomes. Thus, it does not produce a single score, but rather a list of important comorbid conditions a patient has been indicated to have. The Elixhauser method has been shown to outperform the Deyo adaptation of the Charlson comorbidity index for predicting in-hospital mortality in patients with myocardial infarction.[7]

■ Assessing Risk

Descriptive analysis and simple statistical testing allows for comparison of risk factors between groups and is the first step to making adjustments to risk. Side-by-side comparisons of treatment groups to compare the frequency (percent) or means of important risk variables is the first step to understanding how great the differences are between patients in the study. Simple statistical tests can be performed to determine if differences between risk factors are likely due to chance (not significant) or are significantly different and may have an impact on interpretation of results. If there are no meaningful differences between any known demographic or clinically relevant variables, risk adjustment may not make a substantial difference in results.

To assess risk, it is also important to compare the outcomes of interest in predefined subsets of patients that are known to vary in risk. An example would be to compare costs and benefits in mutually exclusive subgroups of patients of increasing age. A stratified analysis of hypertensive patients may compare cardiovascular outcomes in patients stratified by different levels of patients' blood pressure at the start of the study. It is also common to see outcomes stratified by different levels of risk indices, such as the Charlson comorbidity index described previously.

When comparing outcomes across stratified groups of patients, a few observations can be made. First, whether the outcomes are indeed poorer as risk strata increase. Using the previous example: Do older subgroups have worse outcomes than younger? Do patients who have higher blood pressure at baseline have poorer outcomes, and do outcomes worsen as blood pressure increases? If this is true, these factors may bias treatment comparisons if they are not balanced across treatment groups.

■ Adjusting Risk

Multivariate Analysis

The most common method of adjusting for patient differences is the application of **multivariate analysis**. This statistical method, also referred to as **regression**

analysis, is designed to measure the independent contribution of multiple factors to differences in an outcome. This is a very powerful method, because it allows for simultaneous correction of risk factors to produce risk-adjusted estimates of outcomes and treatment group differences. Although the details of this statistical approach are beyond the scope of this chapter, multivariate techniques such as ordinary least squares regression and logistic regression are common methods employed in outcomes studies to correct for selection bias.

The association between each factor included in the regression and the outcome of interest is simultaneously measured. The treatment group is included with all other risk factors, so that the association between treatment and outcome can be measured while correcting for the effects of all other variables in the analysis. Results of multivariate analysis applied to treatment groups are often described as the difference between treatments, after controlling for all other factors included in the analysis.

In addition to regression analysis, one should consider whether the differences observed between groups are consistent at different levels of risk. If one treatment group is clearly better than another at all different levels of risk, there is greater indication that a difference between treatments is real. Likewise if the difference is inconsistent, or if there is no difference between groups at different risk strata, the evidence of association between treatment and outcome is poorer.

Propensity Scores

The **propensity score** method is a statistical technique that overcomes these limitations by combining multiple differences in patient characteristics into a customized score that can be used for risk adjustment.[8] The idea behind the propensity score is to use as much of the data that is available about a patient *prior* to receiving treatment to predict the likelihood of a patient to receive one treatment or another. A score between 0 and 1 is calculated for each patient that represents the likelihood of being in one treatment or another, based on differences in patient characteristics. One treatment group will have patients with scores closer to 0; the other will have patients closer to 1. For example, if treatment group 0 has a lower proportion of female patients in it than treatment group 1, a female patient will likely have a lower propensity score than an otherwise identical male.

In the process of calculating a propensity score, multiple patient factors that make two treatment groups different are now summarized into a single measure. Factors that are similar between the groups have little impact on the propensity score, whereas factors that are much different between the groups have a large impact. Therefore, the method automatically includes differentiating factors for correction, making the technique efficient.

The calculated propensity scores can then be used to identify and compare patients with similar characteristics. The traditional method involves dividing the total sample into five equally sized subgroups and comparing treatment groups in a stratified analysis. Within each strata of propensity score, patients are typically well-balanced between treatment groups by relevant factors. Across patient subgroups, characteristics often differ, with the greatest differences between the subset with the lowest and highest propensity scores.

Propensity scores can also be used to match patients. Randomly matching patients based on a narrow range of propensity score can be an effective method of obtaining two similar samples for comparison. Because patients are matched by the likelihood of being in one treatment or the other, the **matched samples** will be artificially comprised of patients equally likely to be in one treatment or another. This is similar to the concept of randomization, and the final result is treatment groups that look very much like those randomized to treatment. Comparisons can be made between the matched samples as if they were similar.

Although appealing in concept, there are some limitations to matching. First, there is a limit to how many variables can be matched in two groups. The greater the number of factors, the less likely it will be to find matches. Continuous variables, such as age, must often be summarized to categorical groups in order to create a good match. Finally, matching can drastically reduce the number of patients in an analysis. If matching a single patient in one group to a single patient in another, the maximum sample size is limited to the number of patients in the smaller group. However, this method is increasing in popularity for reducing the bias in comparisons of treatments using large observational datasets.

Instrumental Variables

For risk adjustment to achieve its intended goal—elimination of selection bias— all relevant risks must be properly measured and accounted for in the adjustment. This is difficult, if not impossible, because of all the factors that can influence both treatment selection and outcome. The currently available methods of measuring risk factors are typically well validated for the risks they attempt to measure; however, there are important risk factors that are very difficult if not impossible to observe or measure. A typical risk factor that is difficult to measure is motivation to comply with treatment. This factor may have a large impact on the treatment chosen and on the ultimate outcome of treatment, but the assessment of this factor is typically not done and if it is, it is often imprecise. The advantage of randomization as a design strategy is its ability to correct for both observed and unobserved risk factors. This adjustment for unobserved risk factors is not possible in traditional risk adjustment models.

An **instrumental variable** (IV) is an observable factor that influences treatment choices but does not directly affect patient outcomes.[9] Although there would be a correlation between an instrumental variable and outcome, it is assumed that this correlation is due solely to its influence on treatment choice and not due to a causal relationship between the IV and the outcome. Because of the instrumental variable's relationship to treatment choice, an IV can be used to mimic randomization of patients to a likelihood of being in different treatment groups. When a valid IV is identified and used in the analysis, the resulting estimates of treatment effects are not contaminated by selection bias.

A valid IV is one that acts in a way that determines treatment status in a nondeliberate random fashion. Two conditions are required for validity. First, the IV must not be directly or indirectly correlated with the outcome variable. Second, the IV must strongly influence the probability of receiving treatment. If an IV is identified, comparison of outcomes in treatment groups by the presence of the instrumental variable will provide an estimate of treatment effect that controls for both observed and unobserved patient characteristics.

▮ Time Adjustment

Another adjustment that must be made to data in economic evaluation, that is not at all related to risk or selection bias, is correction for the effects of time on costs and health outcomes. People clearly prefer to receive money and health benefits as early as possible. If offered a choice between $100 today or $100 in 5 years, any rational person would prefer to have the money today rather than wait for it. By having money today, you can enjoy its benefit today, whereas your likelihood of benefiting from money far in the future is uncertain and the benefit you would receive is delayed. The same is true for health, in that people prefer to have health improvement sooner rather than later. These are important factors to consider when comparing treatments that have costs and outcomes that are realized at vastly different points in time.

Discounting is a method employed to reduce the value of monetary and health outcomes over time, such that the further in the future the cost or outcome occurs, the less value that cost or outcome has. The most standard method of discounting is to reduce the value or a future outcome by a specific percentage for each year into the future it occurs. This percentage is called the **discount rate**. A discount rate of 3 percent is often recommended, although rates from 3 to 7 percent are commonly used in studies. During each future year a cost or outcome is multiplied by a discount factor, calculated as follows:

$$\text{Discount factor} = 1 \div (1 + \text{Discount rate})^{\text{Years ahead}}$$

When the equation is applied to costs using a 3 percent discount rate, the following discount factors would result: 1.00 for year 1 (no discounting), 0.971 in year 2, 0.943 in year 3, 0.915 in year 4, and so forth. In Table 5-2, a treatment that costs $15,000 in year 1, and $5,000 for each following year for 5 years is presented. In Table 5-3, calculation of discounted life years is presented in a patient who survives 3.5 years from a treatment. Notice the difference in the final undiscounted and discounted costs and life years. This difference becomes greater as time in the future is increased.

It is recommended that any study of greater than 1-year duration apply a discount rate to future costs and outcomes. The most common practice is to apply the same discount rate to costs and outcomes. Thus, if a 3 percent discount rate is chosen in a cost-utility analysis, both costs and QALYs from each treatment would be discounted at this rate, and the cost-effectiveness ratio would be the ratio of the difference between the sum of discounted costs and QALYs of treat-

Table 5-2 Discounting Future Costs

Undiscounted and discounted costs of an initial $15,000 cost followed by $5,000 per year for 4 years, using a 3% discount rate.

Costs by Year ($)	Undiscounted Cost ($)	Discounted Cost ($)
Year 1	15,000	15,000
Year 2	5,000	4,854
Year 3	5,000	4,713
Year 4	5,000	4,576
Year 5	5,000	4,442
Total	35,000	33,585

Table 5-3 Discounting Future Life years

Undscounted and discounted life years calculated for an individual surviving 3.5 years, using a 3% discount rate.

Survival by Year	Undiscounted Life Years	Discounted Life Years
Year 1	1.00	1.00
Year 2	1.00	0.97
Year 3	1.00	0.94
Year 4	0.50	0.46
Total	3.50	3.37

ments under study. Because there is no universally accepted discount rate to use, long-term studies commonly report results using one predefined rate as their primary analysis, and then also report the results using lower and higher rates to demonstrate the impact of discounting on the conclusions of the study.

It is important to note that discounting is independent from **inflation**. When calculating costs in economic analysis and prior to discounting, costs must be recorded in a common currency year. If the study has collected historical costs over several years, costs from the past can be expanded to current dollars by multiplying them by an inflation rate. If the study is extrapolating costs in the future, such as costs predicted from a long-term model, simply using cost estimates from the current year is sufficient to correct for the effects of inflation. Discounting would then be applied to future costs as explained earlier.

Conclusions

Several adjustments must often be made in economic evaluations to make results valid and relevant for public policy decision making. Failure to apply appropriate adjustments can result in incorrect conclusions about more cost-effective treatments. Economic evaluation can be very challenging, particularly when the data from which the analysis is conducted is drawn from sources with different patient types and health systems.

There is no perfect means to correct for selection bias other than randomization. Even the best adjustment will be hindered by natural limitations in data quality and the inability to correct for unknown, unmeasured, or unmeasurable risk factors. The interaction between risk factors can be infinitely complex and impossible to distinguish without truly balanced patient samples achieved through good randomization. However, randomized studies take a long time, are very expensive, and are often unable to recruit patients who represent the vast population in which a treatment is received. Therefore, observational studies will continue to be a primary component of economic evaluation, and risk-adjustment methods will continue to be developed and refined to improve the validity of these critical economic comparisons.

Despite the limitations, economic analysis is very important, and the best attempt should be made to make accurate and reliable comparisons of treatments. By measuring risk, applying the best methods to correct for risk, and correcting for the effects of time, fair comparisons between treatments are possible. Continuing economic evaluations can occur as more data is collected and better quality trials can be conducted if necessary.

Case Study

Consider the objective of assessing whether coronary catheterization is a cost-effective procedure following acute myocardial infarction (AMI). Due to the intensity of this intervention and its perceived benefit, randomization to receive catheterization is not possible. However, many sources of data may be used to compare this treatment from an observational setting

Data from Medicare beneficiaries who had an acute myocardial infarction are available over a 5-year period. Data includes demographics, comorbid disease, incidence and date of death, zip code, and all charges for healthcare services for at least 1 year prior to and 4 years following the initial AMI admission. For each hospital where treatment was received, hospitals may be classified based on the frequency of performing catheterization procedures and volume of AMIs in elderly patients in the year. The outcome of interest is long-term cost-effectiveness of catheterization following an AMI.

Consider the following:

1. What comparison will be made to determine the value of coronary catheterization?
2. What factors may affect a 4-year survival in patients who have AMI?
3. What are some factors that may affect the use of catheterization in patients following AMI?
4. What are some risk factors that can be measured in these patients?
5. Should discounting be applied? If yes, how would costs and outcomes be discounted?

Study/Discussion Questions

1. What is a risk factor and how do risk factors affect comparisons between treatments?
2. Describe two methods to measure the risk of poor outcomes from comorbid disease in a cohort of patients.
3. A recently developed treatment for severe pulmonary disease has received limited use, despite having excellent clinical data. You are working with a managed care plan to study the costs and outcomes of patients who receive this treatment compared with patients who do not using their data. Other than costs and outcomes following treatment, what other factors do you need to measure in these patients? What patient factors other than the new treatment could affect the outcomes in patients who are selected to receive the new treatment?

4. A vaccine has been developed that will prevent infection with HIV. A randomized clinical trial has demonstrated that the vaccine is 100 percent effective and has no side effects—however, the cost is quite high, at nearly $500 per administration. Your local health department is considering immunizing every child between the ages of 14 and 16 with this vaccine, but would like your recommendation about the cost-effectiveness of such an intervention. What factors must you consider in making this recommendation?

Suggested Readings/Web Sites

Iezzoni LL, eds. *Risk Adjustments for Measuring Health Care Outcomes*. 3rd ed. Chicago: Health Administration Press; 2003.

References

1. Kaplan MH, Feinstein AR. The importance of classifying initial co-morbidity in evaluating the outcome of diabetes mellitus. *J Chronic Dis*. 1974;27(7-8):387–404.

2. Charlson ME, Pompei P, Ales KL, MacKenzie CR. A new method of classifying prognostic comorbidity in longitudinal studies: Development and validation. *J Chronic Dis*. 1987;40(5):373–383.

3. Deyo RA, Cherkin DC, Ciol MA. Adapting a clinical comorbidity index for use with ICD-9-CM administrative databases. *J Clin Epidemiol*. 1992;45(6):613–619.

4. D'Hoore W, Bouckaert A, Tilquin C. Practical considerations on the use of the Charlson comorbidity index with administrative data bases. *J Clin Epidemiol*. 1996;49(12):1429–1433.

5. Romano PS, Roos LL, Jollis JG. Adapting a clinical comorbidity index for use with ICD-9-CM administrative data: differing perspectives. *J Clin Epidemiol*. 1993;46(10): 1075–1079; discussion 1081–1090.

6. Elixhauser A, Steiner C, Harris DR, Coffey RM. Comorbidity measures for use with administrative data. *Med Care*. 1998;36(1):8–27.

7. Southern DA, Quan H, Ghali WA. Comparison of the Elixhauser and Charlson/Deyo methods of comorbidity measurement in administrative data. *Med Care*. 2004;42(4): 355–360.

8. Rubin DB. Estimating causal effects from large data sets using propensity scores. *Ann Intern Med*. 1997;127(8 Pt 2):757–763.

9. Newhouse JP, McClellan M. Econometrics in outcomes research: the use of instrumental variables. *Annu Rev Public Health*. 1998;19:17–34.

Chapter 6

THE INDUSTRY'S INVOLVEMENT IN ECONOMIC EVALUATION

Dennis M. Meletiche, PharmD
Feride H. Frech, MPH, RPh
Laura T. Pizzi, PharmD, MPH

Overview

In this chapter, we discuss the involvement of manufacturers in the conduct and dissemination of economic evaluation. The rationale for manufacturer interest in economic evaluation is described, as well as how firms typically organize resources involved in performing this type of research. We also discuss the context of economic evaluation in relation to the drug development process; specifically, what type of evaluation is appropriate during both pre- and post-marketing phases. Finally, we discuss issues related to the practical application of economic evaluation by healthcare decision makers, and provide guidance for manufacturers on ensuring the quality and credibility of their work in this area.

Learning Objectives

1. To understand the factors stimulating manufacturers' interest in economic evaluation of drugs and other healthcare interventions
2. To describe the different phases of clinical research and application of economic evaluation during each phase
3. To understand how manufacturers may increase the quality and credibility of the economic evaluations they complete

▌Keywords

Clinical development
Formulary
Internal business partners
Lifecycle
Preclinical development
Phase I research
Phase II research
Phase III research
Phase IV research

▌Introduction

Over the last decade, economic evaluations have become increasingly important to the manufacturers of healthcare interventions—especially pharmaceuticals—as a means of determining the value of new products. As a result, health economics and outcomes research (HEOR) departments have emerged within small firms and were expanded within larger manufacturers. These departments are responsible for conducting research on the economic aspects of drug products versus treatment alternatives. In addition, they perform cost or burden of illness studies to determine where the sources of cost for specific diseases or medical conditions. The research efforts are typically aimed at determining the value of specific products to healthcare providers, patients, and payers (the latter including private insurers, state and federal government, and large employers).

The involvement of manufacturers in economic evaluation has sparked an ongoing debate as to whether or not it is ethical for the makers of healthcare interventions to be performing economic evaluations involving their products.[1] Furthermore, there is question as to whether it is appropriate for manufacturers to use such evaluations in promotional efforts. Supporters of industry involvement in economic evaluation argue that companies investing in such research will reap the rewards of better market access and product commercialization,[2] though this should not occur at the expense of good scientific practices. In contrast to clinical research, where bias is often easy to identify, bias in economic evaluation may be unrecognizable. This is because the quality of such evaluations hinges upon the breadth and depth of data incorporated into the analysis, as well as the appropriateness of calculations made. Healthcare decision makers are becoming more adept at critiquing such studies and it is in the manufacturer's best interest to adhere to scientific principles when performing economic evaluations.

▌ Why Are Manufacturers Interested in Economic Evaluation?

Market pressures represent the primary reason why the manufacturers of drugs and other healthcare interventions are interested in performing economic evaluations. In an attempt to control rising healthcare expenditures, the payers and providers of health care in this country—namely, the government, large hospitals/health systems, and managed care insurers—often implement specific measures to ensure the appropriate utilization of healthcare interventions. These techniques are perhaps best exemplified by the case of pharmaceuticals, in which the utilization of drug products is managed using a **formulary**. The concept and operation of formularies is further discussed in Chapter 7. In brief, formulary management may involve

1. requirement of prior authorization for payment of certain drugs or unusual dosages;
2. limits on the quantity of product dispensed; and
3. tiered copayments, in which patients are required to pay less for cheaper medications (e.g., generic medications) and more for expensive brands.

Because these utilization controls may have a significant impact on the commercial success of a healthcare intervention, manufacturers must convince payers and providers of the clinical and economic value of their products in order to secure a favorable product positioning.

A second reason for manufacturer interest in economic evaluation is the U.S. Food and Drug Administration's (FDA) activities related to (1) the approval of economic claims regarding drugs and (2) the oversight of promotional materials containing economic data. With respect to economic claims, there is still much debate and lack of clear guidance from the FDA regarding what level of evidence is considered sufficient to substantiate economic claims involving a specific product.[3] A reasonable approach might be to follow the requirements for clinical claims, which is that any such claim made to an *individual prescriber* may be supported by data from at least two randomized controlled trials. Given that economic evaluations typically involve less rigorous types of studies (e.g., retrospective database analyses or nonrandomized trials) and require some level of estimation and/or modeling, manufacturers seldom attain the level of evidence required to substantiate economic claims. As a result, manufacturers currently have limited ability to disseminate the results of an economic evaluation to individual prescribers.

Manufacturers do have more latitude, however, when it comes to sharing economic data to large healthcare insurers and provider organizations. The Food and Drug Administration Modernization Act of 1997 does allow manufacturers to disseminate economic information to formulary decision makers when requested, even if the data are generated from less rigorous types of studies. However, as discussed in Chapter 6, the manufacturer must provide this data in response to an unsolicited request from the organization.

▇ Economic Evaluation in the Context of Product Development

The type of economic evaluation performed by a manufacturer involving a specific product typically varies depending on what stage the product is at in its **lifecycle**. The lifecycle of a product ranges from preclinical development to clinical development (Phases I–III of clinical research), and finally to Phase IV research involving marketed products. Research that occurs prior to human testing is typically called **preclinical development**, which involves testing the drug in laboratory animals or creating computer models to simulate the effect of the new treatment. Economic evaluation during the preclinical phase is typically aimed at determining the cost or burden of illness and consideration of whether there is opportunity for the new intervention to reduce the costs associated with the targeted disease.

In the United States, **clinical development** usually consists of three phases of testing in humans (Phases I–III):

- **Phase I research** trials involve a small group of healthy participants and are designed to determine the drug's pharmacology, pharmacokinetic profile, safe-dosage range, and safety and tolerance in human beings. These trials, which usually last a few months, help establish a safe-dose range and identify any side effects related to the study medication. Economic evaluation during this stage may include development of models to estimate the impact of the new intervention based on preliminary efficacy and safety characteristics. However, some manufacturers may not conduct economic evaluations in Phases I and II because of the limitations associated with the trial design.
- **Phase II research** trials, designed to test the efficacy of the new treatment, involve a larger group of human participants. This is the first study in which affected volunteers (rather than healthy volunteers) are tested. Phase II trials are usually randomized and blinded to ensure objectivity and may require up to 2 years for completion.
- **Phase III research** trials are similar to Phase II trials but at a larger scale, involving hundreds (or even thousands) of human participants. These trials allow much more information to be collected concerning the intervention's safety and efficacy and require a significant time investment (several years). The goal is filing a new drug application (NDA) to the FDA if Phase III trials demonstrated the product to be both safe and efficacious. Data required for economic evaluations, such as direct and indirect costs related to the treatment, is often collected as a part of a Phase III trial. In such cases, economic

end points are typically secondary to gathering safety and efficacy data and are said to be gathered "alongside" of the clinical trial. The utilization of healthcare services and productivity losses (presenteeism and/or absenteeism) are usually captured during the clinical trial, then later converted to a dollar value.

- **Phase IV research** is conducted during the postmarketing period of the product lifecycle.

During this postmarketing phase, HEOR departments focus on performing and sharing economic evaluations with specific healthcare payers or providers and may accumulate additional economic data via Phase IV clinical trial and stand-alone studies. Customizable cost-effectiveness models might serve as a useful means of estimating the outcome of treatment alternatives within specific payer or provider organizations. Budget impact models are also useful in cases where payers and provider organizations are interested in understanding the budgetary impact of choosing one treatment alternative versus another.

Economic evaluation is an evolving field, as is the organization of HEOR departments within drug and device manufacturers. One of the published surveys on the composition and organization of such departments was conducted in 1998 by a group of investigators at the Center for the Study of Drug Development at Tufts University.[4] Respondents included HEOR directors from 45 different pharmaceutical companies. The investigators used 1996 annual sales as the criterion to classify the companies as small (sales less than US $3 billion), medium (sales between US $3 billion and US $7 billion), or large (sales in excess of US $7 billion). At that time, HEOR departments had only been in existence for an average of 6 years. Larger companies had a longer history with a formalized HEOR function and also employed more than twice the number of full-time staff devoted to economic evaluation (mean of 16.9 Full-time equivalent) compared to medium- and small-size companies. The majority of respondents anticipated a substantial expansion of their departments in the following 2 to 3 years, indicating a corporate commitment to economic evaluation and recognition of its value.

Companies with HEOR functions differ in terms of whether such research falls under research or marketing operations. In the United States in particular, there is increased government scrutiny on the marketing practices of pharmaceutical companies resulting in a clear trend toward greater separation between research and marketing activities. This separation is intended to minimize the potential for commercial influence on industry-sponsored research—including economic evaluations. This trend may affect the reporting structure of HEOR departments, with a majority likely to be housed under research operations.

It is important to recognize that HEOR researchers within the industry do not work in isolation. Individuals from multiple departments in the firm, also known as **internal business partners**, provide input relevant to the planning and execution of economic evaluations. The departments or functional areas that regularly collaborate with HEOR departments include the clinical development, marketing department, regulatory affairs, and statistics. It is important to recognize that these departments may have different names in different companies, but the role and responsibilities and their interaction with HEOR should be fairly similar across different firms:

- The marketing department provides the commercial context for the planning of economic evaluations. For example, they help HEOR understand prescribing trends as indicated by market share of drugs and collaborate in the determination of the relevant perspective for the evaluation based on the expected customers (i.e., employers, managed care organizations, or the government).

- The regulatory affairs department ensures that HEOR activities comply with internal policies as well as external legal and regulatory requirements (the most relevant of which is Section 114 of the FDAMA), provides input on how the results of economic evaluations may be disseminated (e.g., in promotional materials), and advises HEOR researchers on the filing of economic claims with the FDA.

- The clinical development department collaborates with HEOR researchers when economic end points are included in clinical trials. Typically, a representative from the clinical development department is primarily responsible for the execution and general oversight of the trial, while the HEOR representative ensures that the appropriate economic variables and costing methodology are used. Medical directors also provide guidance on the design of stand-alone HEOR evaluations (such as selection criteria identifiable with ICD-9-CM codes when conducting an economic evaluation using retrospective claims database analysis).

- Statistics departments frequently collaborate with HEOR personnel in cases where an economic evaluation involves more sophisticated data analyses or must be completed using a specific type of statistical software.

The Sophistication of Economic Evaluations: A Gap between Theory and Practice

Although it's clear that economic evaluation plays a role in determining the value of pharmaceuticals and other treatment interventions, the sophistication of such evaluations may hinder their usefulness in the real world of healthcare decision making. In 1998, Evans and colleagues surveyed a group of medical and pharmacy directors at managed care organizations across the United States on the use of economic evaluation in the formulary decision-making process.[5] The majority of respondents (95%) felt that they had "at least adequate understanding" of the economic evaluation of drugs, vis à vis pharmaceoconomics. However, when respondents were asked about their understanding of common concepts in economic evaluation (such as quality adjusted life years and Markov models), the majority (over 85%) were not familiar with such terms.[5] Furthermore, research by Doubilet and colleagues warned of the misinterpretation of the term *cost-effective*, which is routinely confused in the literature with the term *cost-saving*.[6] These findings suggest that many healthcare decision makers do not understand the science behind economic evaluation, though they comprehend more straightforward economic measures such as drug costs.

In another study, Grabowski and associates assessed pharmacy benefit managers' (PBMs) use of manufacturer-sponsored cost-effectiveness analyses.[7] They interviewed representatives from five major U.S. PBMs and found that such evaluations were of little use in aiding formulary decision making. Specific limitations included:

1. the selection of inappropriate interventions for inclusion in the evaluation,
2. the study population was not relevant to their setting,
3. there were perceived methodological flaws,
4. concerns surrounding the objectivity of industry-sponsored economic evaluations, and
5. the lack of company sales representatives who were able to articulate the relevance of economic findings to their specific PBM firm.

Consequently, it is vital for economic evaluations conducted by manufacturers to be transparent in reporting the methods as well as the data sources used. Such transparency facilitates its customization by any healthcare payer or provider for their own population. Guidelines on evaluating economic analyses endorse such transparency.

In summary, there is presently a gap between the scientific theories surrounding economic evaluation and their use in practice. Manufacturers, as well as any other organization that performs an economic evaluation must address this gap in order to ensure that the target audience of the evaluation, understand the implications of choosing one intervention versus another. One way that manufacturers have attempted to address this gap is by employing field-based scientists who work directly with healthcare payers and providers to both perform and understand the results of economic evaluation.

Industry-Sponsored Economic Evaluations: Ensuring Quality and Credibility

In 1999, Gagnon published one of the best practical reviews of the key elements of an industry-sponsored economic evaluation.[8] In his review entitled "What

Constitutes a Useful Health Economic Study for the Pharmaceutical Industry?" Gagnon synthesized the literature on how managed care, pharmacy, and industry representatives view the application of economic evaluation in decision making. Based on input from this group of stakeholders, Gagnon compiled a list of the characteristics of what he called a "useful" economic evaluation. These characteristics could be categorized into four critical elements (see Figure 6-1):

1. Credible
2. Transparent
3. Timely
4. Comprehensive

Economic models, in particular, have been criticized for lack of objectivity and transparency. Olson and colleagues conducted a survey that resulted in recommendations regarding how to improve the usefulness of industry-sponsored economic models.[9] Those surveyed included 20 research scientists who worked for pharmaceutical and biotechnology companies, but were responsible for presenting economic models to managed care organizations. Results revealed factors that contribute to the success of an economic model:

Figure 6-1 Characteristics of the Ideal Economic Evaluation

1. Credible
   - Published in a peer-reviewed journal
   - Performed by credible researchers
   - Based on good-quality medical evidence
   - Based on credible data sources
   - Consistent results in different patient populations
   - Results tested with sensitivity analysis
   - Available in publications that decision makers read
   - Disseminated by industry representatives with expertise in health economics

2. Transparent
   - Detailed description of data sources
   - Disclosure of all assumptions

3. Timely
   - Need to start health economic evaluation early in the development of the drug
   - Results must be available in time for pharmacy and therapeutics committee review

4. Comprehensive
   - Incorporates all comparators for treating illness
   - Incorporates head-to-head comparisons with competing products
   - Measures the impact of the drug on total health system costs, hospital length of stay, reduction in hospitalization, patient productivity (for employers), and other end points used by decision makers

Source: Adapted from Gagnon J. 2003. What Constitutes a Useful Health Economic Study for the Pharmaceutical Industry? *American Heart Journal,* 137(5)628–665, Copyright (1999) with permission from Elsevier.

1. The model is presented to a small audience of decision makers that includes both physicians and pharmacists
2. The presenter is credible (can fully explain the model and understands the needs and priorities of the audience)
3. The model is simple and transparent in terms of how calculations are made
4. It may be customized using the population characteristics and costs from individual managed care organizations
5. The content of the model is credible and sources are referenced
6. Reprints of publications(s) on the model are made available

In general, industry-based researchers may enhance the credibility of their studies by partnering with both reputable academic investigators and clinicians who care for the population of interest and publishing their findings in credible peer-reviewed journals. Researchers should use data sources that are widely accepted in the research community, and when possible, directly applicable to the target population. Repeating the same study in various populations and obtaining consistent results would further strengthen the credibility of any economic evaluation. Finally, sensitivity analysis should be performed to test the robustness of results.

Conclusion

The manufacturers of healthcare interventions often use economic evaluation as a tool to assist decision makers in understanding the value of different treatment alternatives. Although the conduct of such studies by manufacturers is sometimes perceived as biased, market forces have resulted in a thirst for economic evaluation on the part of healthcare decision makers, which has been met, at least to some extent, by manufacturers.

The organization of economic evaluation resources (HEOR groups) within a manufacturing firm differs, with some functioning under marketing/commercial operations, and others functioning under research operations, moving forward, it is expected that, with a trend toward greater separation between research and commercial activities, that HEOR groups will operate as research entities.

Manufacturers complete different types of economic evaluations during different stages of product development. Early on, during Phase I research, manufacturers engage in cost or burden of illness studies in order to understand the major cost drivers associated with the disease of interest. Later during development, manufacturers may collect actual economic data during clinical trials or develop economic models based on the findings from clinical trials. Models are also useful during the postmarketing phase, particularly if they can be customized to suit the needs and interest of specific payer and provider organizations.

Given their direct stake in the success of a product, it is essential for manufacturers to adhere to good scientific practices when performing economic evaluation. This includes considering all relevant data and ensuring transparency in terms of how calculations are made. Manufacturers may further enhance the quality and credibility of an economic evaluation by involving academics who specialize in economic evaluation, as well as clinicians who care for patients receiving the interventions of interest.

Because manufacturers typically possess what healthcare payers and providers often don't—namely, the resources and expertise to perform sound economic evaluation—they hold the opportunity to advance the state of knowledge and application of such evaluations within the broader healthcare community.

▌ Case Study

The following case study describes how a pharmaceutical manufacturer could use a budget impact model to help a state Medicaid system assess the potential impact of adding a new product to their formulary.

Due to extremely tight budgets, state Medicaid systems are under tremendous pressure to contain healthcare costs. Mental health costs, in particular, pose a formidable challenge to Medicaid administrators. There is high prevalence of mental health conditions in the Medicaid population and it has been documented that these patients utilized more health services than patients without mental health conditions. Antidepressants represent the most commonly prescribed agents in this population and are also the largest budget item in the pharmacy budget.

A pharmaceutical manufacturer is launching a new antidepressant called Vaderal. This new product exerts its pharmacological effects through a different mechanism of action from previously released competitors. The available clinical data suggest that Vaderal is safe and effective in treating major depression. Although there are no head-to-head studies with the major competitors, the available data indicate that Vaderal may have a similar efficacy and safety profile. The average wholesale price for Vaderal is 5 percent lower than the least expensive of the currently available antidepressants, making it the least expensive agent.

Because there are no evident clinical differences between Vaderal and the competing agents, the manufacturer may decide to focus on its lower acquisition cost as the main argument to gain formulary placement on the state Medicaid system. A budget impact model focused exclusively on antidepressant cost would be a simple, yet highly effective way to highlight the magnitude of potential savings to Medicaid. The model would allow Medicaid to utilize their utilization data to determine their current expenditures on the antidepressant class. The model would also allow the user to assess how potential changes in market share from more expensive agents to Vaderal will translate into savings for Medicaid. What practices would be useful for ensuring the quality of the model? What presentation strategies might the manufacturer use to make the model more understandable to Medicaid payers?

Study/Discussion Questions

1. What type of evaluation is appropriate during both pre- and postmarketing phases?
2. Is there bias in economic evaluations?
3. What are the strengths and weaknesses of using economic evaluations?

Suggested Readings/Web Sites

Anderson KM, Bala MV, Weisman HF. Economics and cost-effectiveness in evaluating the value of cardiovascular therapies. An industry perspective on health economics studies. *Am Heart J.* 1999;137(5):S129–S132.

Centers for Medicare and Medicaid Services. Available at: www.cms.hhs.gov/statistics/nhe/historical/chart.asp. Accessed January 10, 2005.

Hughes DA, Walley T. Economic evaluations during early (phase II) drug development: A role for clinical trial simulations? *Pharmacoeconomics.* 2001;19(11):1069–1077.

Sloan FA, Whetten-Goldstein K, Wilson A. Hospital pharmacy decisions, cost-containment, and the use of cost effectiveness analysis. *Soc Sci Med.* 1997;45(4):523–533.

References

1. Drummond MF. A reappraisal of economic evaluation of pharmaceuticals science or marketing? *Pharmacoeconomics.* 1998;14(1):1–9.
2. Thwaites R, Townsend RJ. Pharmacoeconomics in the new millennium a pharmaceutical industry perspective. *Pharmacoeconomics.* 1998;13(2):175–180.
3. Neumann PJ, Claxton K, Weinstein MC. The FDA's regulation of health economic information. *Health Aff.* 2000;19(5):129–130.
4. DiMasi JA, Caglarcan E, Wood-Armany M. Emerging role of pharmacoeconomics in the research and development decision-making process. *Pharmacoeconomics.* 2001;19(7):753–766.
5. Evans CE, Dukes EM, Crawford B. The Role of Pharmacoeconomic Information in the Formulary Decision-Making Process. *J Manag Care Pharm.* 2000;6(2):108–121.

6. Doubilet P, Weinstein MC, McNeil BJ. The use and misuse of the term "cost-effectiveness" in medicine. *N Engl J Med*. 1986;314(4):253–256.

7. Grabowski H, Mullins CD. Pharmacy benefit management, cost-effectiveness analysis, and drug formulary decisions. *Soc Sci Med*. 1997;45(4):535–544.

8. Gagnon JP. What constitutes a useful health economic study for the pharmaceutical industry? *Am Heart J*. 1999;137(5):S62–S66.

9. Olson BM, Armstrong EP, Grizzle AJ, Nichter MA. Industry's perception of presenting pharmacoeconomic models to managed care organizations. *J Manag Care Pharm*. 2003;9(2):159–167.

Chapter 7

FORMULARY DECISION-MAKER PERSPECTIVES: RESPONDING TO CHANGING ENVIRONMENTS

Alan Lyles, ScD, MPH

Overview

Both public health and formularies have a population focus—identifying clinical needs, establishing priorities among these needs and, increasingly, developing optimal policies to produce the greatest impact from limited resources. By adopting a population focus, and basing formulary decisions on their impact on the total system rather than only the pharmacy budget, Pharmacy and Therapeutics (P & T) Committees can improve the quality of pharmacotherapy and enhance the value obtained from resources devoted to pharmaceutical products.

The P & T Committee sets the policies and procedures by which a formulary is developed, managed, enforced, and revised. The Academy of Managed Care Pharmacy (AMCP) Format for Formulary Submissions is an instrument of the P & T Committee that can be used to make a comprehensive dossier of clinical and economic information on pharmaceutical products under its review.

There are a variety of challenges that face formulary decision makers, including technical, business, and ethical issues. Formulary decisions have responded to changing environments that have different requirements and targeted different audiences. The decision-making process now goes through four major stages: *Stage I: Professional Inventory Management; Stage II: Information; Stage III: Restriction;* and *Stage IV: Choice.*

This chapter examines the origins, evolution, and functioning of the formulary process, with an emphasis on the role of economic evaluation.

Learning Objectives

1. To identify key drivers of pharmaceutical and device manufacturer's decisions
2. To learn about the barriers to implementation of economic evaluation
3. To identify organizations inherent to the decision process of economic evaluation

Keywords

AMCP format
Consumer-driven health plans
Evidence-based medicine
Food and Drug Administration Modernization Act of 1997
Formulary
Heroic Co-payments
Incentive
Omnibus Budget Reconciliation Act of 1990
Pharmacy and therapeutics committee
Pharmacy benefit management companies
Pharmacoeconomics
Perscription drug benefit
Point-of-service
Rebates
Reference case
Spread pricing
Stratified formularies
Technology assessment
Tiered or stratified formularies

Introduction

From its origins as primarily a means of inventory and quality control to implementing scientific drug use policies and insurance benefits, the complexity and role of the formulary process have increased substantially. The **formulary** itself is essentially a list of pharmaceutical products; however, it is the most tangible evidence of a pharmacy benefit and, as such, it links physicians, their patients, benefit managers, health insurance purchasers, and health plans. The emergence and expansion of prescription drug insurance benefits for large patient populations have made the differences in their financial interests explicit. Resolving these interests with the limited resources available for insurance benefits has added economic evaluations to the formulary process. Economic evaluations, however, are not conducted in isolation; they are part of a larger system of practices intended to influence and improve medical therapy.

Controlling prescription drug costs in managed care organizations (MCOs), health plans, and pharmacy benefit management companies generally poses both technical and business challenges. The technical challenge is to determine whether the clinical and economic evidence justifies a particular product's being added to a formulary, or covered benefit, and if it does, under what circumstances. The business challenge is to design a benefit package that offers sufficient choice to be attractive to consumers without producing cost increases that require prohibitive insurance premiums or creating perverse incentives such as underutilization of prescription drugs for medication-sensitive conditions. Conversely, high patient cost sharing coupled with a modest **prescription drug benefit** can selectively discourage the enrollment of persons with chronic illness—an alternative approach to restraining medication costs, but one at odds with addressing societies' healthcare needs.

Both public health in the broad context and formularies have a population focus: identifying clinical needs, establishing priorities among these needs, and increasingly, developing optimal policies to produce the greatest health improvements from limited resources. To do this, formulary decision makers must consider the composite, not just the individual impact of their decisions and the global (rather than solely the pharmacy consequences). Economic evaluation is increasingly used to supplement the clinical evidence used by formulary decision makers to determine what place, if any, a drug has in the treatment of the population(s) treated under a particular formulary. However, understanding the current state of formulary decision making and the role of economic evaluation requires a brief historical perspective.

▊ The Evolution of Formulary Management: A Historical Perspective

Over the past 30 years, eight trends have converged to make economic evaluation a practical consideration in formulary decisions:

1. The shift of a large portion of the financial responsibility for prescription drugs from many individuals to large organizations
2. The growing financial liability this represents for those organizations
3. The negotiating power achieved by these organizations
4. The cumulative impact of clinical epidemiology, small-area variation studies, and evidence-based medicine

5. Advances in cost-effectiveness analysis and pharmacoeconomics
6. The development of a cadre of professionals trained in the economic evaluation of pharmaceutical products
7. Advances in information systems that link medical service and pharmacy utilization to provide timely data for economic evaluations
8. The emergence of de facto standards of a formulary system and of the format for clinical and economic information to support that system

Shifting Financial Roles

Formularies increased in importance as prescription drug insurance benefits and the availability of medications grew. Under fee-for-service indemnity insurance, prescription drugs were an infrequent and negotiated benefit. According to the Centers of Medicare and Medicaid (CMS), in 1960, individuals paid out of pocket for 96 percent of prescription drug expenditures, with private health insurance representing just 1.3 percent and public funds 2.7 percent. By 1985, individuals still paid over 55 percent of these expenditures out of pocket, but private health insurance had grown to 29.9 percent and public funds to 14.6 percent. By 1996, however, third parties (private insurers and public programs) accounted for two thirds of prescription drug payments in the United States.[1]

An early competitive advantage of managed care was its coverage of prescription drugs, a benefit that was generally not included in indemnity policies; in 1996, 98 percent of health maintenance organizations (HMOs) offered a prescription drug benefit.[2] HMOs typically offered both lower premiums and some prescription drug benefit, making managed care an attractive option that was generally less costly than indemnity insurance. As employers and insurance purchasers looked to control their outlays for medical expenses, this combination had strong appeal. The Health Maintenance Organization Act of 1973 provided additional incentives to create and to offer HMOs as alternatives to indemnity insurance, but this initial stimulus was feeble because the enabling regulations were only slowly issued.[3]

However, HMO enrollments increased an astounding 793 percent in just 19 years, from 9 million people in 1980 to over 81 million in 1999; between 1990 and 1995 alone there was a 54 percent increase.[4] According to a national survey on the topic, MCOs' formulary goals were to provide appropriate therapy, to provide drug information, and to decrease costs. Additional but less frequently cited goals were to decrease duplication and to control drug use.[5] To meet these objectives, MCOs assess the safety, clinical effectiveness, cost of treatment and cost-effectiveness of pharmaceutical products. A variety of sources for information are used to perform these evaluations: industry data, peer-review literature, government reports, and miscellaneous sources. In the survey, evaluations performed by industry received lower MCO ratings for quality, validity, and comprehensiveness, but the highest for timeliness and availability—resulting in a score for overall importance in drug decisions only slightly below the peer-review literature and well above government reports.[6] What does this tell us about economic evaluation as part of the MCO formulary process? That there is an urgency to these decisions, that they often must be made with incomplete or less valid information, but that they will be made and all sources will be considered, with adjustment for perceived validity by information source. Unfortunately, it also indicates an availability bias—the importance of less-valid information sources is inflated by its timely availability. Taken together, these results suggest suboptimal drug formulary decisions due to information that is delayed, missing, incomplete, or from a biased source.

Looking to the future, surveyed MCOs were willing to use pharmacoeconomic assessments from an external source if these assessments were standardized, readily accessible, and more directly relevant to the drug decisions faced by the organization. However, due to differing perspectives or purposes for the analysis, some experienced difficulty applying the results of an external analysis to the decision(s) in their particular organization. Conversely, internally prepared assessments had greater acceptance and were more frequently considered in drug adoption decisions.[5]

Financial Liability for Prescription Drugs

Managed care enrollments and annual health insurance premium increases moved in opposite directions from 1989 to 1996; premiums slowed from an 18 percent annual increase in 1989 to 0.8 percent in 1996.[7, 8, 9] The annual cost increase per capita for prescription drugs was at its lowest (5.2%) in 1994, but annual drug cost increases experienced double-digit percentages for all but 2 years during 1991 to 1997.[10] Drug expenses increased disproportionately to other categories of healthcare expenditures. Thus, declines in premium revenue growth during periods of overall annual inflation in the range of 2.4 percent to 4.9 percent meant that health plans and MCOs had to manage utilization and expenses aggressively to maintain profitability; their costs for goods and labor, and particularly for prescription drugs, were exceeding premium growth.[8]

In 1995 and 1996, annual per-capita prescription drug spending grew 10.6 percent and 11 percent, while the annual changes in spending for *all* services during the same period were 2.2 percent and 2.0 percent.[11] In order to compensate for these increases in prescription drug costs, health expenditure categories had to decrease even more. MCOs, health systems, and PBMs turned to both utilization controls and financial approaches to influence prescription drug use. Utilization controls included pharmaceutical product selection (such as through closed formularies and/or product exclusions) and/or utilization management initiatives (such as profiling prescribers and prior authorization); financial approaches emphasized benefit design (such as closed formularies), tiered coinsurance formularies, and purchasing incentives (such as mail-order prescriptions for patients and negotiated price discounts for plans). Ironically, the prescription drug cost trend occurred despite continuing problems of inappropriately low adherence and underutilization of prescription drugs for existing medical needs; it is likely that a number of the insurance premium projections and calculations actually incorporated this underutilization.[12] This process unfortunately encouraged a compartmentalized management structure—one that manages and rewards performance by individual service silos or categories. Under silo management, product price, utilization, and line item budgets dominate; and possible costs of increased utilization in one sector (such as pharmaceuticals) versus offsets in another (such as emergency or institutional care) are passively if not actively discouraged.

Negotiating Power

Growing managed care enrollments and agressive contracts for companies that manage pharmacy benefits provided the size and purchasing power for MCOs to obtain price concessions from manufacturers. At the same time, organization around provider networks for defined patient populations provided the structure to apply their data in order to influence drug-use patterns. Additionally, their financial accountability for pharmaceutical product use provided the motivation to do so.

Although MCOs consider the financial impact of formulary decisions, they have the option of determining which costs are relevant to their decisions: "hard costs" such as products with short expiration periods or high risk for being discarded, and "soft costs" such as personnel costs incurred in product preparation, handling, and administration frequency. For example, Carolinas HealthCare System weighed precisely these factors in their decision on whether to change from a third-generation cephalosporin (an antibiotic) to a then-recently available generic cephalosporin product similar in spectrum and therapeutic applications. In that instance, "soft dollar" costs and intangibles such as anticipated patient satisfaction due to less frequent dosing led to a decision not to change, demonstrating that direct costs are not the sole determinant when more complete information is available and a system impact framework is adopted.[13]

The Buyers Health Care Action Group (BHCAG), an employer group purchasing initiative in Minneapolis–St. Paul, determined that its early experience with a centralized formulary was incompatible with the decentralized delivery system that it had organized around competing independent care systems. Consequently, BHCAG contracted with a PBM to provide each care system with technical support and assist in formulary development consistent with the care system's provider and patient profiles. Formulary adherence was to be achieved by a combination of tailored formularies that met clinical requirements and return of negotiated rebates not to BHCAG but to the independent care systems.[14]

Pharmacy benefit management companies (PBMs) are another key stakeholder in formulary decisions. PBMs arose from the obscurity of claims processing and mail-order pharmacy services to become multibillion dollar companies. They accomplished this through acquisitions, leveraged purchasing power, and expertise providing expanded clinical and management services to MCOs, employers, and insurers to control prescription drug costs. PBMs achieve efficiencies and competitive advantage by accumulating contracts with numerous clients to "carve out," or manage under contract, the pharmacy component of a health insurance benefit.[15] Organizations adopt a carve-out strategy because they lack the expertise or infrastructure required to manage a particular service area. PBMs focus nearly exclusively on drug costs—a classic instance of silo management—and only recently have begun to expand to other services such as disease management. In this way, PBMs achieved economies of scale in their core administrative functions, but they also realized substantial negotiating power to obtain lower product prices from manufacturers. PBMs offer a full range of pharmacy management services and formulary options, but it is the client's decision as to which to use. The PBM business model is based on service fees for administering the pharmacy benefit, providing mail-order services and developing formularies.

Some PBMs rely on a two-stage decision process: (1) the **pharmacy and therapeutics** (P&T) **committee** (either within the PBM or outsourced) to assess medications for safety, efficacy, and placement against the current formulary listings; and (2) if the new product poses no therapeutic advantage over an existing product, then it is treated as a commodity with its cost negotiated accordingly and the formulary placement being determined by the best negotiated price among the substitutes.[16]

A PBM also earns revenue through **rebates**. These are payments from pharmaceutical manufacturers based on the PBM's achieving negotiated market-share levels for specific drug products. Formulary construction for PBM clients ultimately includes contractual relationships between PBMs and the drug manufacturers in which incentives and rebate arrangements are made explicit. Some PBMs fully discuss rebates with their clients; however, these arrangements are not generally disclosed to the PBM's clients and this led to concerns over effective discharge of the PBM's fiduciary responsibilities—first, regarding less than complete disclosure of the portion of the rebate retained by the PBM versus what is paid to the client, and second, whether the specific products recommended by the PBM are in their client's best financial interest or if they are selected because they provide a larger rebate to the PBM.[17] **Spread pricing** occurs when the payment to the pharmacy is less than what is billed to the client for that product reimbursement; hence, the "spread" creates an additional margin for the PBM.[18, 19]

Writing in 1997, Grabowski reported that PBMs did not use cost-effectiveness analyses (CEAs) extensively in making formulary decisions, but they did have the data and the informational infrastructure to support such analyses. PBMs' reluctance to use CEA was based on concerns that the then-existing studies had no, or the wrong, comparator; reported on populations dissimilar to those served by the PBM; came with an extensive list of methodological restrictions; and/or had a perceived lack of objectivity due to funding source. Consequently, PBMs asserted that formularies determined on the basis of price (less rebates) were cost saving for a health plan and were justified until cost-effectiveness was adequately demonstrated. Specifically, they requested economic evaluations that featured head-to-head comparisons among market leaders, studies performed on relevant populations, timely availability of information, independent sponsorship or "no-strings" funding, publication in leading peer-reviewed journals, and more sophisticated drug representatives who can discuss nuances of a study.[16]

Evidence-Based Decisions

Increased drug use and costs did not mean that the best value was being obtained for these payments. Rather, from the early 1970s, epidemiological data demonstrated large variations in the rate of medical services and procedures between small contiguous areas, even when the underlying medical need was similar in the communities being compared.[20, 21, 22] These small-area variations of several-fold differences (and more) have been replicated across clinical disciplines, geographical settings, patient populations, and time. More recently, Motheral demonstrated similar regional variations in prescription drug use, both on a per-capita basis and for specific products.[23]

The durability of these variations suggests that training or local practice norms may have more influence on prescribing behaviors than a systematic and scientific review of the evidence would support. There is pervasive underuse of basic recommended pharmacotherapy in routine ambulatory medical practice that "poses serious threats to the health of the American public,"[24] including medications essential for managing serious chronic diseases such as asthma, cardiovascular disease, congestive heart failure, diabetes mellitus, coronary artery disease, and mild or uncontrolled hypertension. This growing body of evidence led purchasers to demand **evidence-based medicine** that would base medical practice on the systematic identification, appraisal, and synthesis of clinical studies, particularly randomized clinical trials.[25] A P&T committee's evidence-based decisions, pharmaceutical use policies, and educational outreach can influence and potentially reduce variations to those resulting mainly from patient differences. "In an increasingly complex clinical care delivery environment, [the goal should be to] structure care delivery so that evidence-based best practice is the default course."[26]

A summary of the peer-reviewed literature demonstrates that purchaser demands for evidence of value resulted in an explosion of health economic publications. Reviewing the trends in cost-benefit analyses (CBAs) and CEAs from 1979 to 1996, Elixhauser and associates identified 3,539 studies that included both costs and consequences.[27] The largest increases in published studies were for pharmaceutical products and occurred during 1991 to 1996 (years that overlapped the dramatic growth of managed care enrollments). As numerous authors reported during and after this period, the published results were of uneven rigor, unstandardized methodologies and frequently indistinguishable from marketing materials—leading one author to describe **pharmacoeconomics** as "a pseudodiscipline . . . conjured into existence by the magic of money."[28] Sloan noted that ". . . in the private sector . . . formal analysis of costs and benefits does not appear to be widespread," nor did it appear that economic analyses were being performed routinely within organizations to assist their own decisions.[29]

As P&T committees grappled with evidence-based formulary decisions, the impact of the Prescription Drug User Fee Act (PDUFA) in expediting reviews of new drug applications complicated their work.[30] From 1993 to 1995, the FDA averaged 25 approvals per year for priority and standard new molecular entities (NMEs) combined. The first full impact of PDUFA in reducing the median review time for new drug applications produced 53 NME approvals in 1996 and an average of 34.7 over the next 3 years.[31] These faster review times, however, resulted in P&T committees having fewer published studies available when their decisions on a new product's comparative economic and clinical profiles and its formulary status had to be made.

Access to information on off-label drug uses and economic communications concerning pharmaceutical products are governed by FDA regulations. Although this information may allow for a more comprehensive product evaluation, doing so requires the decision maker to have appropriate training and expertise to judge correctly the cumulative significance of the evidence presented. A P&T committee's expertise in evaluating the credibility and value of diverse sources of product information is recognized by the FDA under the **Food and Drug Administration Modernization Act** (FDAMA) **of 1997**.[31] The FDAMA authorizes pharmaceutical manufacturers to communicate directly with P&T committees regarding off-label information (Section 557) and health economics and modeling studies that meet certain criteria (Section 114). To regulate promotional activities, however, the FDA requires that the P&T committee must first make an unsolicited request to the manufacturer for this information.[32, 33]

WellPoint Pharmacy Management is taking the next step in pharmaceutical product assessment by addressing gaps in their information dossier through targeted studies using WellPoint's members. WellPoint's outcomes–based formulary addresses two shortcomings of existing information sources—dossier information deficits and dissimilar groups studied versus enrolled in the plan(s). The WellPoint National Pharmacy and Therapeutics Committee uses the results of these targeted studies when reviewing possible formulary product changes.[34]

Methodology Employed in Economic Evaluations

The profusion of economic impact studies did not, however, resolve the P&T committee's needs for rigorous studies using objective criteria. The main factors that continue to limit the use of economic evaluations are their variability and relevance to the P&T decisions; particularly with respect to the analyst's choice of[35]:

1. Time frame
2. Discount rate
3. Analytic perspective (societal, individual, firm, or plan)
4. Treatment of indirect costs
5. Accuracy, relevance, and completeness of direct costs
6. Protocol generated costs and/or cases
7. Treatment of endpoints
8. External validity of the study sample
9. Sample size
10. Statistical power

Standardizing the treatment of these factors seems reasonable, even obvious, but it has not yet occurred. No individual or group has been able to specify the information requirements or methodology in sufficient detail to render economic evaluations directly useful to formulary decision makers. Beyond the specifications, there is the residual challenge of motivating producers and consumers of this information to adhere to such a format voluntarily.

Australia has been an early leader in national evidence-based prescription drug decisions and its experience with the Australian Pharmaceutical Benefits Scheme (APBS) suggests a steep learning curve, both for those preparing the guidelines for submission and for those submitting economic evaluations in support of a product. Sixty-seven percent (67%) of a sequence of 326 submissions to the APBS were determined to have "serious problems of interpretation," such as the estimated comparative clinical efficacy, the comparator product(s) selected for the analysis, the models, and even calculation errors.[36]

Over the last 15 years, however, there have been methodological advances in the application of economic evaluations and a series of initiatives by major stakeholders to define a structure that would address these shortcomings for formulary decision makers. To appreciate the appropriate role and use of economic evaluation by P&T committees, it is essential to place current practice(s) in the context of evolving free-market initiatives, where advances have taken hold, largely as a result of meeting the demands of decision makers.

Seeking to establish standards for CEA that would lead to more reliable information for policy decisions, the U.S. Public Health Service convened the Panel on Cost-Effectiveness in Health and Medicine in 1993. After two and a half years, the panel produced a widely cited set of recommendations in its final report: "Cost-Effectiveness in Health and Medicine."[37] The panelists acknowledged that no one approach or set of assumptions would be able to meet the legitimately different needs of stakeholders who produce and who use CEA results. Because CEA results performed under differing assumptions might not be directly comparable, they recommended reporting a **reference case** for each that would allow such a comparison. The reference case would consist of "a standard set of methodologic practices that an analyst would seek to follow in a cost-effectiveness study" in addition to analyses where the CEA analyst's requirements depart from the reference case assumptions.[37] This recommendation is a substantial methodologic contribution, but there has not been widespread adoption of it in practice.

Over the next 5 years there were more attempts to close the gap between the decisions required of P&T committees and ensure that relevant information is available when formulary decision(s) had to be made. In 1995, the Pharmaceutical Research and Manufacturers of America (PhRMA) proposed voluntary guidelines for health plans.[38] The following year, Langley and Sullivan proposed a therapy intervention framework for assessing population health outcomes and total health system impact of pharmaceutical products, rather than solely the pharmacy budget impacts.[39]

In a subsequent proposal to Blue Cross and Blue Shield of Colorado and Nevada, Langley proposed a more comprehensive solution: basing formulary decisions about pharmaceutical products on standard drug dossiers; evidence-based criteria, using a systems impact framework; and producing transparency in the assumptions and calculations in the manufacturer's economic model(s).[40] In this way, the baseline and subsequent changes in resource use associated with a proposed formulary addition could be modeled using a plan's own data.

Regence BlueShield, a health plan in the Northwestern United States, was also striving to make formulary decisions based on demonstrated value rather than price or promotional incentives. Their approach has had a national impact. Regence's guidelines provided: (a) more timely access both to published and to unpublished studies, off-label use information, humanistic, and economic studies; (b) a disease rather than a drug-based model to assess a product's impact on the whole Regence system; and (c) a standardized dossier submitted by the manufacturer, thereby reducing the time required for Regence's clinical pharmacists to assemble the product summary for the P&T committee. Regence's initiative was successful, in part, because it was the largest regional health plan and 45 percent of its pharmacy plans relied on a closed formulary.[41] The Academy of

Managed Care Pharmacy (AMCP) subsequently developed and disseminated an adaptation of Regence's approach to meet the needs of health plans and PBM formulary decision makers, although this standardized process of reporting clinical and economic information is just the beginning.[42, 43]

Training in Economic Evaluation

Unfortunately, the applications of CEA to pharmaceutical product evaluation(s) preceded broad-scale training of pharmacy professionals and other decision makers in these techniques. In a 1995 survey, 92 percent of a nationally representative sample of HMOs reported that they would use drug assessments from an external source, but only 65 percent were familiar with assessments that used modeling.[44] The difference suggests that even well-done analyses may not be distinguishable from poorly performed ones without additional training for MCO staff. P&T committee members were expected to incorporate economic evaluations into their decisions, yet, most did not have formal training on the topic. Although articles explaining the methods of economic evaluation and checklists for reviewing related articles had appeared in the literature, texts by Drummond and Bootman provided a pivotal framework for practitioners.[45, 46]

Since then, economic evaluation techniques have become an established component of pharmacy and public health curricula, and may also be learned through a fellowship program. These sources can now be supplemented by continuing education courses and, more recently, by AMCP training activities. In addition, targeted publications such as *P&T Committee* and *Formulary* are available, which address issues from the P&T committee's perspective. General publications such as the *American Journal of Managed Care, Clinical Therapeutics, Pharmacoeconomics, The International Journal of Technology Assessment in Health Care, Health Services Research,* also now now carry timely peer-reviewed reports relevant to economic evaluation.

Integrated Data

The pressure for integrated linked medical service and pharmacy utilization data for members of managed care plans increased as the plans grew in size. In the private sector, provider and insurer demands for evidence from economic evaluations stimulated the growth of contract research organizations that specialized in pharmaceutical products and health technology assessment. They and other organizations developed proprietary databases that may be purchased by researchers performing economic evaluations of drugs. In some cases these data may include laboratory utilization, which can be used to complete economic evaluations of diagnostic tests. However, these databases are not equally appropriate for the range of economic evaluation questions that may be posed.[47]

Standards

Clinical and economic information that are timely, complete, unbiased, and relevant to the formulary process are the most basic requirements for making decisions that influence drug product use in patient populations. This has been elusive; however, an emerging de facto standard format adopted by health plans, PBMs, and government programs is being advanced by the AMCP.[43, 48]

The **AMCP Format** provides a template for clinical and economic information concerning a product being considered for formulary inclusion. The format specifies in detail both the process and a standardized dossier of information to be exchanged between drug manufacturers and P&T committees (see Appendix A). AMCP prepared its format to assist health plans in initiating their own unsolicited requests for a standard set of clinical and economic information. Unlike the formulary review of a pharmaceutical product that typically would have been compiled by an MCO or contracted third party, the AMCP Format primarily relies on the manufacturer to provide the information.[34] This comprehensive template may be particularly useful to smaller organizations or those with fewer resources for assembling complete drug dossiers for P&T committee reviews. The format encourages economic models that[42]

1. are transparent and interactive (to be useful for formulary decisions);
2. produce results relevant to the organization's formulary decisions;
3. provide an audit trail;
4. present uncertainty in the model parameters and their estimates through sensitivity analyses; and
5. provide results that can subsequently be transferred to drug reviews and monographs.[42]

The requested economic model is open; that is, it is not secured, hidden, locked, or otherwise inaccessible to decision makers. With an open economic model, one can examine the logic behind the decision rules and, if they are satisfied with it, they can adapt the analysis to their own plan. For example, they can replace the manufacturer's data with their own population-specific cost and utilization characteristics. The P&T committee is hence released from the constraints posed by closed, or locked, models that have sometimes been used in the past. Additionally, decisions based on models for newly released products can be reexamined after the plan accumulates its own experience with the product.[49] Finally, the format does not specify the type of economic evaluation to be used—only that it be performed at the level of thoroughness expected of professional practitioners.

The Formulary Process

The formulary itself is an intermediate step in the larger process of supporting rational pharmacotherapy and value-based decisions. The membership of the P&T committee and the policies and procedures by which the formulary is managed, are critical to achieving these results.

The P&T committee is responsible for managing the formulary system. It is a multidisciplinary group composed of physicians, pharmacists, and other health care professionals with expertise in pharmaceuticals. Its responsibilities include developing and revising the formulary, establishing policies on the use of formulary and nonformulary pharmaceutical products, and educational activities to support scientific pharmacotherapy.

Formulary Varieties

In the ambulatory setting, formularies are most often linked to insurance benefits; consequently, there are different types to support different insurance products. They vary in how they attempt to influence specific drug choices and the extent of patient cost sharing or participation required in the decision. Typically, prescription cost-sharing is less for on-formulary, or preferred products, and greater for off-formulary or nonpreferred products.

The main formulary types are *open, closed, negative,* or *incentive based.* An *open* formulary does not pose barriers to the use of a pharmaceutical product, although it may indicate or only list preferred agents. A *closed* formulary, by contrast, only includes agents that have met the P&T committee's inclusion criteria and prescription drug insurance benefits are restricted to that list, except in specified instances. *Partially open* or *partially closed* (or *negative*) formularies selectively include or exclude classes or products.[50]

By adopting a population focus and basing formulary decisions on their impact on the total system rather than only the pharmacy budget, P&T committees can improve the quality of pharmacotherapy and enhance the value obtained from resources devoted to pharmaceutical products. In the hospital setting, the P&T committee historically consisted of respected local community practitioners representing multiple disciplines and working toward consensus, similar to institution review boards or ethics committees. Peer representation, coupled with evidence-based decisions and the opportunity for practitioners to present their case for a product, support the committee's authority and the acceptance of that authority by the prescriber.[51]

Increased formulary use in the 1990s and an anticipated Medicare pharmaceutical benefit based on one led seven national organizations in 2000 to develop the Core Principles of a Sound Drug Formulary System.[52] Collectively, these principles enhance the likelihood that formulary decisions will support the clinical needs of patients while operating within the pharmacy benefit. The principles concerning economic considerations are provided in Table 7-1.

Formulary decisions require the P&T committee to have a thorough understanding of a pharmaceutical product's strengths and limitations; a process for assessing the product's clinical and economic profiles relative to competing products and the morbidity patterns of the covered populations; and an objective assessment of the most likely impact a therapeutic change will have on the population(s) served.

Accreditation Criteria

Accrediting bodies have formal criteria for medication management by the organization or plan undergoing accreditation review. The Joint Commission on Accreditation of Healthcare Organizations (JCAHO) implements medication management standards in a variety of organizations, including ambulatory care, behavioral health, hospital, home care, and long-term care facilities. Although it began and is largely known for its work in establishing standards and accrediting hospitals, JCAHO made medication management a priority focus area for 2004.[53]

Table 7-1 Economic Considerations Under the Principles of a Sound Drug Formulary System

1. Assess peer-reviewed medical literature, including: randomized clinical trials (especially drug comparison studies), pharmacoeconomic studies, and outcomes research data.
2. Base formulary decisions on cost factors only after the safety, efficacy, and therapeutic need have been established.
3. Evaluate drug products and therapies in terms of their impact on total health care costs.
4. Permit financial incentives only when they promote cost management as part of the delivery of quality medical care; financial incentives or pressures on practitioners that may interfere with the delivery of medically necessary care are unacceptable.
5. Require P&T committee members to reveal, by signing a conflict of interest statement, economic and other relationships with pharmaceutical entities that could influence committee decisions.
6. Exclude product sponsor representatives from P&T committee membership and from attending P&T committee meetings.
7. Require P&T committee members to adhere to the formulary system's policy on disclosure and participation in discussion as it relates to conflict of interest.
8. Inform physicians, pharmacists, other health professionals, patients, and payers about the factors that affect formulary decisions, including cost containment measures; the procedures for obtaining nonformulary drugs; and the importance of formulary compliance to improving quality of care and restraining healthcare costs.
9. Provide the rationale for specific formulary decisions when requested.

The seven organizations in the coalition that developed the principles are: The Academy of Managed Care Pharmacy, the Alliance of Community Health Plans, the American Medical Association, the American Society of Health-System Pharmacists, the Department of Veterans Affairs Pharmacy Benefits Management Strategic Healthcare Group, the National Business Coalition on Health, and the U.S. Pharmacopeia.

Source: Reprinted with permission from the Foundation for Managed Care Pharmacy. Web site: http://www.amcp.org/data/nav_content/drugformulary%2Epdf.

Alternatively, HMOs and other healthcare organizations may seek accreditation from the National Committee on Quality Assurance (NCQA), a private, non-profit organization whose focus is the improvement of healthcare quality. The NCQA accreditation standards for pharmaceutical management are designed to ensure that "the organization develops, regularly reviews and updates policies and procedures for pharmaceutical management based on sound clinical evidence." Key elements of NCQA's standards include "(1) the criteria used to adopt pharmaceutical management procedures, and (2) a process that uses clinical evidence from appropriate external organizations."[54] Consequently, economic criteria alone are insufficient for pharmaceutical management systems and procedures.

Stages of Formulary Decision Making

Formulary decisions have responded to changing environments that have different requirements and targeted different audiences. The evolution has not been solely from one stage of development to the next; sometimes they overlap and occasionally a stage may be essentially skipped, but four different functional stages can be identified (Figure 7-1).

Stage I: Inventory

Formularies provide an opportunity to control inventory expense and reduce product duplication. Early hospital-based economic evaluations were essentially limited to cost comparisons and astute purchasing. However, rising hospital costs in the late 1970s led to the application of economic evaluation tools to both pharmaceutical products and clinical services.[55, 56, 57] The subsequent implementation of a prospective payment system for hospitals using case payments based on diag-

Figure 7-1 Evolutionary Stages of Formulary Decision Making

	Theme	Primary Focus
Purpose: Selecting Among Options		
Stage 1: Inventory	Scientific Inventory Control	Professionals
Stage 2: Information	Persuasion and Relative Product Costliness	Professionals
Purpose: Working with Limits		
Stage 3: Restrictions	Insurance Benefit Restrictions and Cost Sharing	Patients
Stage 4: Choice	Demonstrated Value (Economic Evaluations) and Willingness to Pay	Patients

nosis-related groups (DRG) in 1983 was vast, complicated, and clearly changed the management incentives and expectations for hospital pharmacy. Circumstances similar to those supporting economic evaluations in hospitals were experienced subsequently in the ambulatory setting under managed care: financial and clinical responsibility for a defined patient population, options but different costs among the available pharmaceutical products and services, and limited payments rather than cost-plus or fee-for-service reimbursement.[58]

Stage II: Information

The development of economic evaluation methods and their use in pharmaceutical product assessments did not immediately affect health insurance benefits or restrictive formularies. In the ambulatory setting, purchasers and patients had to become more receptive to the practice. In addition, physicians in the early 1990s were still largely autonomous professionals who resisted oversight and what they perceived as intrusions on their prescriptive authority.

As a negotiated benefit, the existence and extent of prescription drug coverage under employment-based insurance has been somewhat dependent on the state of the economy, the unemployment level, and labor negotiations. In periods of low unemployment, generous health insurance benefits are one way to recruit and to retain valuable employees—insurance benefits that restrict choice more than competing employers' offerings may thwart recruitment in a tight employment pool or even result in an exodus of existing employees. Employers are familiar with this balance—as recently as 2002, 44 percent of firms that increased the amount employees paid for their health insurance reported it to be somewhat to much harder to attract and retain qualified workers, compared with 28 percent of the firms that had not increased the amount employees paid.[7, 8]

	Economic Parameters	Clinical Parameters	Quality of Life Parameters
Patients	±	✓	✓✓
Physicians	±	✓	±
Health Plans	✓	✓	±
PBMs	✓	✓	±

Legend
✓ = interested
✓✓ = very interested
± = interested in certain cases

Figure 7-2 Parameters of Interest to Stakeholders in the Formulary Decision-Making Process

Consequently, MCOs, health systems, and PBMs generally began this stage with open formularies. A representative Stage II formulary would be organized by therapeutic drug classes, with subcategories and individual agents in each. Products would commonly be listed by generic name with the brand being included for reference only. These formularies would typically indicate, though not require, the use of preferred pharmaceutical products and, through various icons, the relative costliness of the formulary products. For example, formulary entries may include a rating from one (the least costly) to four dollar signs to indicate the relative costliness of each product within a particular therapeutic subclass. At this stage of formulary development, these economic determinations would more often have resulted from price comparisons than from formal cost-effectiveness analysis.

There was ample evidence that physicians did not have an accurate understanding of the cost implications of the prescriptions they wrote, or did not feel that it was a relevant factor.[59, 60] Communicating the comparative expense of open formulary products was mainly intended as persuasion, to inform prescribers and to encourage their reflection on this cost information before writing a prescription. There is little to demonstrate that this approach was broadly successful or that it had its intended effect. Therefore, the fundamental divergence of patient, physician, health plan and PBM interests continued (Figure 7-2). Over time, additional formulary practices such as step therapy, prior authorization, and generic, and/or therapeutic substitution came to be used in conjunction with economic evaluations and restrictive formularies.

Stage III: Restriction

Managed care's growth altered pharmaceutical product use in fundamental ways:
1. The focus shifted from individuals to patient populations.
2. The number of people with prescription drug insurance benefits increased.
3. Physician prescribing was subjected to more profiling.
4. The selection, procurement, and use of pharmaceutical products came under greater oversight.
5. Physician and patient choices of insured pharmaceutical products were restricted.
6. Generic pharmaceutical use increased.
7. There were more requests of manufacturers for evidence of value or cost-effectiveness of the products being evaluated for possible formulary inclusion.

For manufacturers, providing evidence of clinical efficacy was familiar terrain; however, these changes meant that their products were now expected to compete for insurance coverage on economic criteria.

In 1990 just 44 percent of HMOs reported using a formulary, but by 1999, 97 percent reported using one.[61] According to a 1995 survey, 72.7 percent of plans using a formulary were using an open design, with closed formularies used more often by staff model managed care plans.[2] HMOs' use of closed formularies jumped from 31 percent in 1996 to 48 percent in 1998 and edged to 49 percent in 1999.[61, 62] Despite the leveling of closed formulary use below 50 percent, there was effective product control when closed formularies were used: nearly 90 percent of dispensed prescriptions were for formulary products.[61] In 1999, 71 percent of HMOs still reported allowing a physician to override the formulary, but by 2002, 46.7 percent reported penalizing physicians if they violated pharmacy policy.[63]

The argument on closed versus open formularies pitted cost controls against open access to medications. A 1996 report cited adverse clinical consequences for formularies that restricted open access to pharmaceutical products, though vigorous disagreement over the research methodology and analytic basis of this inference followed its publication—igniting what may have been the first-ever dispute over research methodology actively debated in the popular press.[64] Subsequently, research assessing the elimination of restrictive state Medicaid formularies under the **Omnibus Budget Reconciliation Act of 1990** (OBRA) concluded that it increased access to specific products but that access resulted in limited or no therapeutic gain from most of them.[65]

Formulary decision makers are aware which benefits that rely mostly on financial cost sharing can produce unintended results. The RAND Health Insurance Experiment demonstrated patient price sensitivity to different amounts of prescription drug cost-sharing.[66] A more recent study on the impact of the introduction of cost sharing for prescription drugs on poor patients and those over 65 years of age demonstrated that both essential and nonessential medication use declined, resulting in increased emergency and hospital care use.[67]

Restrictive health insurance benefits, particularly limitations on choice and direct access, resulted in a consumer backlash to managed care by the mid to late 1990s. By 1996, more than 1000 legislative initiatives were filed to regulate HMOs, resulting in 56 laws in over 35 states.[68] To remain competitive, the next evolution of insurance products featured greater consumer choice. These plans, referred to as **point-of-service** (POS) options, typically allowed patients to choose out-of-network providers and/or nonpreferred formulary medications, but at a higher level of cost sharing. Though this type of insurance gained in popularity, it failed to control expenses, motivating the next major innovation in health insurance benefits.

Stage IV: Choice

Consumer-driven health plans were a response to the backlash against managed care's restrictions on choice, point-of-service plans' lack of cost controls, and the need for affordable health insurance premiums. These plans typically consist of a health or medical savings account that the insured uses as first-dollar coverage under a high-deductible health plan. Costs exceeding the savings account are paid through personal funds until a deductible is met; once the deductible is reached, the insurance plan then acts as a major medical option.[69] The rationale for this design is to replace insurer oversight with oversight by the insured themselves. Plan members have a personal financial interest in the cost of their health services under this type of insurance; but, in theory, it is coupled with more information and Web-based tools to support informed personal choices. Although consumer-driven health plans are still a modest portion of all employer coverage, where the plans are in place, substantial generic substitution rates have occurred.[70]

The transition to consumer-driven health plans has been accompanied by movement away from restrictive formularies toward **incentive**, also known as **tiered**, or **stratified formularies**. Three-tier formularies were beginning to be used in the late 1990s but were rapidly adopted from 2000 (27 percent of workers) to 2003 (63 percent).[8] First-tier products are usually generic drugs and have the lowest cost sharing, the second tier includes preferred branded products, while the third tier is for nonpreferred branded products and carries the highest cost sharing—sometimes referred to as requiring **heroic co-payments**. In addition to the differences in patient cost sharing by tier, the average spread *between* the tiers has increased in recent years.[71] In an employer survey, the average copayment for first-tier (generic drugs) was $10 in 2004; $21 for second-tier (preferred products); and $33 for nonpreferred.[9] The principal goals of incentive formulary designs are to shift costs to consumers; to move the MCO, health plan, or PBM member's utilization toward specific products, supporting the plans' negotiating leverage with manufacturers; and to retain more choices for patients and physicians than would have been available under a closed formulary. Patient cost sharing presents a direct cost reduction to the insurer, and possibly other savings, if prescriptions for nonessential medications are unfilled.

An organization's timely access to its own clinical experience and cost profiles can improve the quality of its decisions by systematically focusing on value rather than price. Recent empiric research provides evidence that moderate changes in patient cost sharing implemented sequentially may support greater medication adherence by patients with chronic conditions. Compared to a plan that only changed from a two- to a three-tier formulary, a plan that both changed from a one- to a three-tier benefit and raised member co-payments has a greater likelihood that plan members would discontinue their medications. That plan's members also made drug switches consistent with their co-payment incentives and the plan had slower drug-cost increases but at what cost in excess morbidity and possible greater total cost?[72] A pre- versus post-comparison group study in a PPO examined longer term (30 months) pharmaceutical and medical services utilization following a change to three-tier copayments. In that study, chronic medication use was not significantly different for the conditions studied except for oral contraceptives at the 6-month milestone; hospitalization, emergency, and office visits were comparable between the intervention and control groups, and drug costs were lower in the intervention group as was use of third-tier medications.[73]

While incentive formularies shift costs to patients and encourage more selective use of pharmaceutical products, their focus on the single cost category of pharmaceuticals may result in unintended consequences in the form of increased use of other services such as the emergency room or hospital. Thirty percent of survey respondents in 2002 who had a condition for which a regular prescription drug is indicated, reported not filling their prescription and 21 percent reported using lower than the prescribed dose to extend the duration of the prescription. When out-of-pocket costs exceeded $100, 50 percent reported not filling a prescription and 35 percent reported using a lower than prescribed dose.[74] Recognizing the risk of lower adherence to pharmacotherapy under an incentive formulary, some implementations of this benefit structure offer more complete insurance coverage for medications to treat a list of prespecified chronic conditions. Other medications would then be paid from a patient's personal account.

Consequently, decisions regarding which type of formulary and what evidence should be considered are crucial to effective pharmaceutical product use. Economic evaluations that focus on price exclusively, or that ignore the interdependencies of separately budgeted medical resources, will be less effective.

Summary and Conclusions

Cost pressures on prescription drug benefits will not relent, yet consumers will continue to demand both affordable health insurance premiums and choices in their care. Evidence-based trade-offs are most likely to preserve a prescription drug insurance benefit, retaining access to the medically essential, even if not to the individually desirable.

New directions in consumer-directed, or high-option, benefit plans coupled with incentive formularies are moving beyond the simple distinctions of brand versus generic to value decisions linked to capped coverage limits. Clinical and economic evaluations jointly, though not equally, influence these formulary decisions. Although the AMCP Format is improving the consistency and relevance of the information on which formulary decisions are based, the relative paucity of economic information for newly approved medications means that the use of modeling to *predict* the costs and effectiveness of treatment will increase. Periodic formulary product reviews can then rely more on the individual plan or population's experience with a product.

Economic evaluations were previously possible in principle, but the integrated data and expertise to produce and to evaluate them were not widely available or sufficient to the needs of most MCOs and health plans. However, in recent years, information technology developments, fellowships, academic programs, continuing education and professional societies are reducing those barriers by providing the data and expertise required to conduct economic evaluations.

The trend for insurance products in the United States is for fewer absolute restrictions such as closed formularies; however, this openness forces explicit choices between products and requires patients to make trade-offs based on their own costs. The formulary's central role in implementing these insurance benefits, coverage decisions, and the extent of patient cost sharing challenges the formulary committee's decisions. Formularies will continue to distinguish between vital, affordable medications and optional, more costly ones by shifting more direct costs and selection decisions to the consumer. Because the consumer-driven health plan structure requires patients to participate in medication use decisions, insurance purchasers and patients will demand more transparency and credibility for specific formulary product decisions.

To be effective, however, formulary committees and the organizations they serve must communicate both the clinical rationale and the economic impact for specific formulary products. Currently, even the main facts from thorough, high-quality formulary decisions based on sound evidence are lost to consumers who choose their medications based on their out-of-pocket expense. From the formulary decision makers' perspective, having patients (and physicians) make a choice based solely, or essentially, on price or their cost-sharing amount, is a failure. Decisions that include, but are not limited to price impacts require informed consumers—yet this information is neither routinely available nor used by patients. As patients are presented with greater choice, but at greater out-of-pocket costs, they may be more willing than health plans and insurers to the effectiveness of prescribed treatments with economic considerations.

▌ Case Study

A large MCO with current enrollment exceeding 2 million members is planning to enter the market for Medicare Advantage, the private health plan option under the Medicare Modernization Act of 2003. As part of the MCO's strategy, it plans to include drug coverage using a formulary. In the construction of its formulary, one of the decisions it must make is whether to include a new medication for arthritis, as well as which (if any) of the alternatives among existing products for arthritis treatment. The MCO's current experience with older members is limited—97 percent of its enrollment is under 60 years of age.

Arthritis is an underdiagnosed condition that has a high prevalence. Among Americans with a disability, arthritis or rheumatism is the leading cause (17.5%) of their disability.[75] In a 2002 survey covering 30 states, the prevalence of arthritis diagnosed by a physician ranged from 17.8 percent to 35.8 percent. Women had a higher prevalence of arthritis as did older age groups; in those over 65, the median percentage with doctor-diagnosed arthritis was 55.6 percent.[76] Although an estimated 47.5 million people in the United States have chronic joint symptoms (CJS), 21.7 percent have never consulted with a healthcare provider for treatment of CJS—even though one fifth of them report CJS as limiting their activities.[77] Approximately 56 percent of the increase in healthcare costs from 1987 to 2000 was attributable to 15 conditions, a list that included arthritis. For arthritis, 24 percent of the change was attributable to increased population, but 44 percent of it was due to an increase in the cost-per-treated case and 32 percent was due to a rise in the treated prevalence.[78] Therefore, understanding basic demographic trends, epidemiology, and treatment options will be essential to forecasting accurately the MCO's ability to provide needed medical care within constrained resources.

A range of products is available for arthritis treatment, from transcutaneous electrical nerve stimulation (TENS) to oral tables to injectible medications. As part of the P&T committee's information collection, the Cochrane Collaboration offers relatively current reviews covering nonsteroidal anti-inflammatory drugs (NSAIDs) and disease-modifying antirheumatic drugs (DMARDs). Assume that a new DMARD is expected to be released within the next 6 months and that the MCO must decide which, if any, DMARD will be included in its Medicare Advantage formulary. Consider the following questions:

1. What are the relevant clinical factors and outcomes that this MCO should consider in its formulary decision?
2. What are the available and appropriate costs that the MCO should consider in addition to the pharmaceutical product? Why?
3. What are the data sources for each of the costs and clinical factors in questions 1 and 2? Do you have any concerns about their reliability and validity? What do you do when there is no data for some factors?
4. Are the medical and pharmacy utilization data on the MCO's current enrolled population appropriate for modeling the clinical and economic comparisons for these agents? Why?
5. What types of economic models would be appropriate to assist the P&T committee in making its formulary decision?
6. If a comprehensive economic model is already available from a drug's manufacturer, should the MCO use it? If not, why? If so, what specific features would the MCO want it to have? Why?

7. If you were told that injectable medications are paid under the medical budget but oral products were paid under the pharmacy budget, would that influence your decision? What if the decision was for an indemnity insurance product rather than an MCO plan?

Discussion Questions

1. How might conflicts of interest arise in P&T committee decisions? What is an effective way to deal with them?
2. Explain the main differences between each of the four stages in the evolution of formulary decision making.
3. What is an open model formulary and why is it important?
4. The response to a pharmaceutical product within a population of patients is not absolute; it reflects a distribution of responders, nonresponders, and partial responders. In addition, the results observed during randomized clinical trials, efficacy, are often better than the results obtained in usual community practice, effectiveness. How should this uncertainty and the translation of a product's efficacy to an estimate of its effectiveness be reflected in economic evaluation?
5. What are the specific subpopulations about whom you would want to have additional information or analyses?
6. Why should the model for the formulary decision include both the natural units of service and, separately, the cost of each?
7. Is it possible to communicate the scientific content of this decision to plan members in a way that helps them make cost trade-offs and purchase decisions? Should this be a P&T committee responsibility?
8. Will value-based formulary decisions always result in lower drug costs? Explain.

Suggested Readings/Web Sites

Academy of Managed Care Pharmacy: Format for Formulary Submissions V 2.0. www.amcp.org/data/nav_content/formatv20%2Epdf.

Agency for Healthcare Research and Quality: Evidence-based Practice Centers. www.ahcpr.gov/clinic/epc/.

Bootman JL, Townsend RJ and McGhan WF. *Principles of Pharmacoeconomics.* 2nd ed. Cincinnati: Harvey Whitney Books Company; 1996.

Canadian Coordinating Office for Health Technology Assessment. www.ccohta.ca/entry_e.html.

The Cochrane Collaboration: The Cochrane Library. www.cochrane.org/reviews/clibintro.htm.

Drummond MF, O'Brien B, Stoddart GL and Torrance GW. *Methods for the Evaluation of Health Care Programmes.* 2nd ed. New York: Oxford University Press; 1997.

Oregon Evidence-based Practice Center: Drug Effectiveness Review Project. www.ohsu.edu/drugeffectiveness/.

█ Appendix A: AMCP Format for Formulary Submissions Version 2.1, A Selected Content Summary

*Unsolicited Letter of Request
1. Product Information
    1.1 Product Description
    1.2 Place of Product in Therapy
        1.2.1 Disease Description
        1.2.2 Approaches to Treatment
    1.3 Evidence for Pharmacogenomic Tests and Drugs

2. Supporting Clinical and Economic Information
    2.1 Summarizing Key Clinical and Economic Studies
        2.1.1 Evidence Table Spreadsheets of all Published and Unpublished Trials
    2.2 Outcome Studies and Economic Evaluation Supporting Data
        2.2.1 Evidence Table Spreadsheets of all Published and Unpublished Outcomes Trials

3. Modeling Report
    3.1 Model Overview
    3.2 Parameter Estimates for Models
    3.3 Perspective, Time Horizon and Discounting
    3.4 Analyses
    3.5 Presentation of Model Results
    3.6 Exceptions

4. Product Value and Overall Cost

5. Supporting Information
    5.1 References Contained in Dossiers
    5.2 Economic Models
    5.3 Formulary Submission Checklist

*Available at:
http://www.fmcpnet.org/data/resource/Format~Version_2_1~Final_Final.pdf.

Adapted with permission from the Foundation for Managed Care Pharmacy.

References

1. Centers for Medicare and Medicaid Services. National Health Expenditures, selected calendar years: 1980–2003. Available at: http://www.cms.hhs.gov/statistics/nhe/historical/tables.pdf. Accessed May 25, 2004.

2. Hoechst Marion Roussel. Managed Care Digest Series: HMO-PPO Digest 1996. Kansas City, MO; 1997.

3. Kongstvedt PR, ed. *Essentials of Managed Care*. 4th ed. Gaithersburg, MD: Aspen Publishers; 2001.

4. Centers for Disease Control and Prevention. Health, United States, 2003. Table 132: Health Maintenance Organizations (HMOs) and Their Enrollment, According to Model Type, Geographic Region, and Federal Program: United States, Selected Years 1976–2002. Available at: www.cdc.gov/nchs/data/hus/hus03.pdf. Accessed October 20, 2004.

5. Lyles A, Luce BR, Rentz AM. Managed care pharmacy, socioeconomic assessments and drug adoption decisions. *Soc Sci Med*. 1997;45(4):511–521.

6. Luce BR, Lyles CA, Rentz AM. The view from managed care pharmacy. Data watch. *Health Aff (Millwood)*. 1996;15(4):168–176.

7. Kaiser Family Foundation and Health Research and Educational Trust. "Employer Health Benefits: 2002 Annual Survey Summary of Findings." Available at: www.kff.org/insurance/3251.pdf. Accessed September 13, 2004.

8. Kaiser Family Foundation and Health Research and Educational Trust. "Employer Health Benefits: 2003 Annual Survey Summary of Findings." Available at: www.kff.org/insurance/ehbs2003-1-set.cfm. Accessed September 13, 2004.

9. Kaiser Family Foundation and Health Research and Educational Trust. "Employer Health Benefits: 2004 Annual Survey Summary of Findings." Available at: www.kff.org/insurance/7148/summary/index.cfm. Accessed September 13, 2004.

10. Center for Studying Health System Change. Consumers Face Higher Costs As Health Plans Seek to Control Drug Spending. Issue Brief No. 45, November 2001. Available at: http://www.hschange.org/CONTENT/389/. Accessed September 10, 2004.

11. Center for Studying Health System Change. Tracking Health Care Costs. Data Bulletin No. 25, June 2003. Available at: www.hschange.org/. Accessed September 10, 2004.

12. Lyles A. Medical spending increases, but pharmaceuticals pose a paradox. *Clin Therap 2002*; 24(2):300–301.

13. Mabe DM. Formulary decision-making about cephalosporins with similar therapeutic uses. *Am J Health Syst Pharm*. 2003;60(10 Suppl 1):S12–S15.

14. Christianson JB, Feldman R. Evolution in the buyers health care action group purchasing initiative. *Health Aff (Millwood)*. 2002;21(1):76–88.

15. Lipton HL, Kreling DH, Collins T, Hertz KC. pharmacy benefit management companies. Dimensions of performance. *Annu Rev Public Health*. 1999;20:361–401.

16. Grabowski H, Mullins CD. Pharmacy benefit management, cost effectiveness analysis and drug formulary decisions. *Soc Sci Med*. 1997;45(4):535–544.

17. Harris KE. PBMs Get subpoenas in federal probe, may delve into rebate, drug-switching. *Health Care Fraud*. 2000;4(6):199.

18. Garis RI, Clarke BE. The spread: A pilot study of an undocumented source of pharmacy benefit manager revenue. *J Am Pharm Assoc.* 2004;44(1):15–21.

19. Latanich T. Pharmacy benefit manager "Spread": A reasonable, rational, realistic business practice. *J Am Pharm Assoc.* 2004;44(1):10–11.

20. Wennberg JE, Gittlesohn A. Small area variations in health care delivery. *Science.* 1973;182:1102–1109.

21. Wennberg JE, Gittlesohn A. Variations in medical care among small areas. *Sci Am.* 1982;246:120-134.

22. Dartmouth. Dartmouth Atlas of Health Care. Available at: www.dartmouthatlas.com about.php. Accessed September 9, 2004.

23. Motheral B. Express-Scripts Fact sheet: Regional variation in prescription drug use. Available at: www.expressscripts.com/ourcompany/news/outcomesconference/2001/factsheets/regionalVariation.pdf. Accessed January 4, 2004.

24. McGlynn EA, Asch SM, Adams J, et al. The Quality of Health Care Delivered to Adults in the United States. *N Engl J Med.* 2003;348(26):2635–2645.

25. Ellrodt G, Cook DJ, Lee J, Cho M, Hunt D, Weingarten S. Evidence-based disease management. *JAMA.* 1997;278(20):1687–1692.

26. James B. Quality improvement opportunities in health care—making it easy to do it right. *J Manag Care Pharm.* 2002;8(5):394–399.

27. Elixhauser A, Halpern M, Schmier J, Luce BR. Health care CBA and CEA from 1991 to 1996: An updated Bibliography. *Med Care.* 1998;36(5 Suppl):MS1-9, MS18–147.

28. Evans RG. Manufacturing consensus, marketing truth: Guidelines for economic evaluation. *Ann Intern Med.* 1995;123(1):59–60.

29. Sloan FA, ed. *Valuing Health Care: Costs, Benefits, and Effectiveness of Pharmaceuticals and Other Medical Technologies.* New York: Cambridge University Press; 1995.

30. U.S. Food and Drug Administration. Prescription Drug User Fee Act of 1992, Pub L No. 102–571.

31. U.S. Food and Drug Administration. Approval Times for Priority and Standard NMEs: Calendar Years 1993–2003. Available at: www.fda.gov/cder/rdmt/NMEapps93-03.htm. Accessed September 12, 2004.

32. U.S. Food and Drug Administration. Food and Drug Modernization Act of 1997 (FDAMA). Public Law 105-45. Available at: www.fda.gov/cder/guidance/105-115.htm. Accessed September 10, 2004.

33. Neumann PJ, Claxton K, Weinstein MC. The FDA's regulation of health economic information. *Health Aff (Millwood).* 2000;19(5):129–137.

34. Sweet BT, Wilson MD, Waugh WJ, Hess AD, Spooner JJ. Building the outcomes-based formulary. *Dis Manage Health Outcomes.* 2002;10(8):473–477.

35. Powe NR, Griffiths RI. The clinical-economic trial: Promises, problems and challenges. *Controlled Clin Trials.* 1995;16:377–394.

36. Hill SR, Mitchell AS, Henry DA. Problems with the interpretation of pharmacoeconomic analyses: A review of submissions to the Australian pharmaceutical benefits scheme. *JAMA.* 2000;283(16):2116–2121.

37. Gold MR, Siegel JE, Russell LB, Weinstein MC, eds. *Cost-Effectiveness in Health and Medicine.* New York: Oxford University Press; 1996.

38. Clemens K, Townsend R, Luscombe F, Mauscopf J, Osterhaus J, Bobula J. Methodological and conduct principles for pharmacoeconomic research. Pharmaceutical Research and Manufacturers of America. *Pharmacoeconomics.* 1995;8(2):169–174.

39. Langley PC, Sullivan SD. Pharmacoeconomic evaluations—guidelines for drug purchasers. *J Manag Care Pharm.* 1996;2(6):671–677.

40. Langley PC. Formulary submission guidelines for Blue Cross and Blue Shield of Colorado and Nevada. structure, application and manufacturer responsibilities. *Pharmacoeconomics.* 1999;16(3):211–224.

41. Mather DB, Sullivan SD, Augenstein D, Fullerton DS, Atherly D. Incorporating clinical outcomes and economic consequences into drug formulary decisions: A practical approach. *Am J Managed Care.* 1999;5(3):277–285.

42. Academy of Managed Care Pharmacy. ACMP Format for Formulary Submissions Version 2.1. April 2005. Available at: www.amcp.org/data/nav_content/ formatv20%2Epdf. Accessed May 28, 2004.

43. Sullivan SD, Lyles A, Luce B, Gricar J. AMCP guidance for submission of clinical and economic evaluation data to support formulary listing in United States health plans and pharmacy benefit management organizations. *J Manag Care Pharm.* 2001;7(4):272–282.

44. Luce BR, Lyles CA, Rentz AM. Data watch: The view from managed care pharmacy. *Health Aff (Millwood).* 1996; 15(4):168–176.

45. Drummond MF, O'Brien B, Stoddart GL, Torrance GW. *Methods for the Evaluation of Health Care Programmes. 2nd ed.* New York: Oxford University Press; 1997.

46. Bootman JL, Townsend RJ, McGhan WF. *Principles of Pharmacoeconomics. 2nd ed.* Cincinnati: Harvey Whitney Books Company; 1996.

47. Lyles A. Pharmaceutical economics and health policy research using administrative data. *Clin Therap.* 2004;26(7):1122–1123.

48. Neumann PJ. Evidence-based and value-based formulary guidelines. *Health Aff (Millwood).* 2004;23(1):124–134.

49. Cox ER, Motheral B, Mager D. Verification of a decision analytic model assumption using real-world practice data: implications for the cost effectiveness of cyclo-oxygenase 2 inhibitors (COX-2s). *Am J Manag Care.* 2003;9(12):785–794.

50. Covington TR, Thornton JL. Chapter 4: The Formulary System: A Cornerstone of Drug Benefit Management. In Ito SM and Blackburn S, eds. *A Pharmacist's Guide to Principles and Practices of Managed Care Pharmacy.* Alexandria, VA: Foundation for Managed Care Pharmacy; 1995.

51. Fins JJ. Drug Benefits in managed care: Seeking ethical guidance from the formulary? *J Am Geriatr Soc.* 1998;46(3):346–350.

52. Academy of Managed Care Pharmacy. Principles of a sound drug formulary system. consensus document. October 2000. Academy of Managed Care Pharmacy. Available at: www.amcp.org/data/nav_content/drugformulary%2Epdf. Accessed September 10, 2004.

53. Joint Commission on Accreditation of Healthcare Organizations. A Guide to JCAHO's Medication Management Standards. Available at: www.jcaho.org. Accessed September 9, 2004.

54. National Committee for Quality Assurance: 2004/2005—Standards and Guidelines for the Accreditation of MCOs. Washington, DC. 2004.

55. Bootman JL, Wertheimer A, Zaske D, Rowland C. Individualizing gentamicin dosage regimens on burn patients with gram-negative septicemia: A cost-benefit analysis. *J Pharm Sci.* 1979;68(3):267–272.

56. Bootman JL, Zaske D, Wertheimer AL, Rowland C. Cost of individualizing aminoglycoside dosage regimens. *Am J Hosp Pharm.* 1979;36(6):368–370.

57. McGhan W, Rowland C, Bootman JL. Cost-benefit and cost-effectiveness: Methodologies for evaluating innovative pharmaceutical services. *Am J Hosp Pharm.* 1978;35:133–140.

58. Moon M. *Medicare Now and in the Future.* 2nd ed. Washington, DC: The Urban Institute Press, 1996.

59. Safavi KT, Hayward RA. Choosing between apples and apples: Physicians' choices of prescription drugs that have similar side effects and efficacies. *J Gen Intern Med.* 1992;7(1):32–37.

60. Glickman L, Bruce EA, Caro FQ, Avorn J. Physicians' knowledge of drug costs for the elderly. *J Am Geriatr.* 1994;42(9):992–996.

61. Aventis Pharmaceuticals. Managed Care Digest Series 2001. Parsippany, NJ: Aventis Pharmaceuticals.

62. Aventis Pharmaceuticals. Managed Care Digest Series 2000. Parsippany, NJ: Aventis Pharmaceuticals

63. Aventis Pharmaceuticals. Managed Care Digest Series 2003. Parsippany, NJ: Aventis Pharmaceuticals.

64. Horn SD, Sharkey PD, Tracy DM, Horn CE, James B, and Goodwin F. Intended and unintended consequences of HMO cost-containment strategies: Results from the managed care outcomes project. *Am J Manag Care.* 1996;2:253–264.

65. Walser BL, Ross-Degnan D, Soumerai SB. Do open formularies increase access to clinical useful drugs? *Health Aff (Millwood).* 1996;15(3):95–109.

66. Leibowitz A, Manning WG, Newhouse JP. The demand for prescription drugs as a function of cost-sharing. *Soc Sci Med.* 1985;21(10):1063–1069.

67. Tamblyn R, Laprise R, Hanley JA, et al. Adverse events associated with prescription drug cost-sharing among poor and elderly persons. *JAMA.* 2001;285(4):421–429.

68. Bodenheimer T. The HMO backlash—righteous or reactionary? *N Engl J Med.* 1996;335(21):1601-1604.

69. Gabel JR, Lo Sasso AT, Rice T. Consumer-driven health plans: Are they more than talk now? *Health Aff (Millwood).* Web exclusive 2002;W395-W407. Available at: content.healthaffairs.org/cgi/content/full/hlthaff.w2.395v1/DC1. Accessed September 10, 2004.

70. Dubose J. Health Leaders Research: Reviews Mixed for Consumer-Driven Plans. Available at: www.healthleaders.com/news/feature1.php?contentid=51398. Accessed January 7, 2004.

71. Novartis. Novartis Pharmacy Benefit Report: Facts and Figures. East Hanover, NJ: Novartis Pharmaceuticals. 2002.

72. Huskamp HA, Deverka PA, Epstein AM, Epstein RS, McGuigan KA, Frank RG. The effect of incentive-based formularies on prescription-drug utilization and spending. *N Engl J Med.* 2003;349:2224–2232.

73. Fairman KA, Motheral BR, Henderson RR. Retrospective, long-term follow-up study of the effect of a three-tier prescription drug copayment system on pharmaceutical and other medical utilization and costs. *Clin Therap.* 2003;25(12):3147–3161.

74. Harris Interactive. Higher out-of-pocket costs cause massive non-compliance in the use of prescription drugs, and this is likely to grow. *Health Care News.* 2002;2(22):2.

75. Centers for Disease Control and Prevention. Adults who have never seen a health-care provider for chronic joint symptoms—United States, 2001. *MMWR.* 2003;52(18):416–419.

76. Centers for Disease Control and Prevention. Prevalence of doctor-diagnosed arthritis and possible arthritis—30 states, 2002. *MMWR.* 2004;53(18):383–386.

77. Centers for Disease Control and Prevention. Prevalence of disabilities and associated health conditions among adults—United States, 1999. *MMWR.* 2001;50 (7):120–125.

78. Thorpe, K. E., C. S. Florence, P. Joski. Which medical conditions account for the rise in health care spending? *Health Affairs (Millwood).* 2004;W4-437–W4-445.

Chapter 8

THE U.S. REGULATOR'S PERSPECTIVE IN DETERMINING AND IMPROVING THE VALUE OF HEALTHCARE INTERVENTIONS

Richard G. Stefanacci, DO, MGH, MBA, AGSF, CMD
Jennifer H. Lofland, PharmD, MPH, PhD

Overview

The Food and Drug Administration (FDA) and the Centers for Medicare and Medicaid Services (CMS) play key regulatory roles in guiding decision making in relation to medical treatments. FDA's history and its increasing use of economic evaluation promote a more comprehensive view of drug approval and monitoring, balancing efficacy, safety and cost. CMS' quality improvement initiatives aim to measure and provide data for development and implementation of policies that promote evidence-based care.

This chapter will describe the present and future activities of the FDA and CMS in utilizing economic evaluation to make decisions regarding medical treatments in the United States.

Learning Objectives

1. To identify the role of the FDA and the legislation governing this organization
2. To learn why CMS is reluctant to use economic evaluation to make decisions regarding coverage or reimbursement
3. To understand how CMS currently allocates healthcare resources
4. To understand the role of economic evaluation in CMS' decision-making processes
5. To discuss the application of economic evaluation in the CDC's Vaccines for Children program

Keywords

Certificate of Medical Necessity
Federal Food and Drug Act of 1906
Food and Drug Administration Modernization Act (FDAMA) of 1997
Food, Drug, and Cosmetic Act of 1938
Healthcare Quality Initiatives
Kefauver-Harris Amendments of 1962
Medicare Payment Advisory Commission
Prescription drugs
Prescription Drug User Fee Act of 1992
Vaccines for Children program

Introduction

In the United States, the primary regulatory players are the Centers of Medicare and Medicaid Services (CMS), the Food and Drug Administration (FDA), and state governments (which administer Medicaid and other state-specific healthcare programs). To date, Medicaid decisions are made largely by states; hence, the role of economic evaluation in Medicaid decision making varies from state to state. Some states consider economic data for expensive treatments (such as antipsychotics and nutritional formulas), but other states lack the expertise or resources to incorporate economic evaluation into Medicaid program decisions. For this reason, state-specific activities involving economic evaluation are excluded from this chapter. Rather, we will focus on the CMS and FDA as the two major federal bodies concerned with the topic—as well as discuss the application of economic evaluation by the CDC as a part of vaccine program evaluation.

U.S. Food and Drug Administration

The FDA is the federal agency that is responsible for the regulation of medications, food, and biologics in the United States.[1] Since its inception, the FDA has focused on ensuring the safety and efficacy of new medications and other healthcare technologies. However, with incremental regulatory changes in the 1990s, the FDA has increased its regulatory scope and has become concerned with the use of health economic information to support pharmaceuticals.

History of FDA Drug Regulation

In 1906, *The Jungle* by Upton Sinclair, a novel that vividly portrayed the filthy conditions within the U.S. meat packing industry, was published.[2] By exposing the then-current and horrible conditions, it was the impetus for the passage of the **Federal Food and Drug Act of 1906**. This act, which at the time was administered by the Bureau of Chemistry, stated that drugs could not be sold unless they met the specifications of strength, quality, and purity specified by the U.S. Pharmacopoeia and National Formulary.[2] This act also dictated the primary focus of the FDA, which was to ensure that medications were *pure*; marking the beginning of the modern era of the FDA as we know it today.

In 1937, a pharmaceutical manufacturer created an elixir of sulfanilamide, a new dosage form of this antibiotic. However, the solvent used for the antibiotic was a highly toxic substance, similar to antifreeze.[2] The use of this new product resulted in over 100 deaths, of that a large proportion were children. This tragedy led to the passage of the **Food, Drug, and Cosmetic Act of 1938**, which required manufacturers to demonstrate that not only were all new drugs pure but were also *safe* prior to receiving approval and release to the public.

In 1951, Carl Durham and Hubert Humphrey proposed a set of amendments to the Food, Drug, and Cosmetic Act of 1938. The amendment created and defined the two classes of drugs that we have today: "legend" drugs or **prescription drugs** (which require a prescription) and over-the-counter (OTC) medications (which can be obtained without a prescription).[3]

In the early 1960s, thaliomide, a new sedative, was found to be associated with birth defects in thousands of newborns throughout Europe.[4] Fortunately, the medication had not been approved for use within the United States. In 1962, with the support of Senator Kefauver, amendments to the Food, Drug, and Cosmetic Act were passed to ensure that not only were medications pure and safe but *efficacious* as well.[4] The **Kefauver-Harris Amendments of 1962** state that the *efficacy* of a drug must be proven by "substantial evidence," which includes "adequate and well-controlled trials."[5] For the first time, manufacturers had to demonstrate that a drug actually worked (was efficacious) to the FDA and to the public. The passage of the Kefauver-Harris Amendments resulted in a significant increase in the importance of randomized clinical trials in the FDA drug-approval process.

Since its inception, the drug-approval process has been the center of much political debate regarding FDA reform.[5] For the last 40 years, one of the greatest criticisms of the FDA by political leaders and the public was that the approval process was too lengthy, resulting in a delay in patients' access to new and effective medications.[6] In an attempt to address this issue, legislators passed the **Prescription Drug User Fee Act (PDUFA) of 1992**. This act authorized the FDA to charge the pharmaceutical manufacturers for reviewing their medications. In 1997, these fees were approximately $88 million and were used to train and hire over 500 FDA reviewers.[7] According to the FDA commissioner at the time, Dr. David Kessler, the increased income resulting from this act enabled faster drug application reviews. The General Accounting Office (GAO) reported that the average approval time for new drug applications (NDA) submitted to the FDA in 1987 and 1992 were 33 and 19 months, respectively.[8] Stated Dr. Kessler:

> These improved approval times have been made possible by shortening the time for completion of most first reviews to only 12 months. For the drugs submitted to the FDA in fiscal year 1994, we reviewed and acted upon 96 percent of them on time. In addition the GAO found that by 1994, FDA review and approval times were faster than those in the United Kingdom.[8]

The PDUFA was due to expire in 1997. Therefore, as one way to reauthorize it and to incrementally reform the FDA, the Food and Drug Administration Modernization Act (FDAMA) was passed—which amended the Kefauver-Harris Amendments of 1962.[6] Through FDAMA, the FDA was charged with moving from its traditional role of ensuring the safety and efficacy of healthcare technologies to reviewing health economic information concerning drugs to inform healthcare decision making.

Under Section 114, the FDAMA loosened restrictions on the health claims that pharmaceutical industry could make concerning pharmaceutical products and allowed pharmaceutical manufacturers freedom to make economic claims concerning their products.[7]

The FDA and Economic Evaluation

The FDAMA became law in February 1998. However, despite a scheduled release date of May 21, 2002, the FDA has yet to provide interpretative guidance on the use of economic claims (Section 114) in promotional material that is provided to healthcare professionals and patients.[9]

Even though the FDA has not provided definitive guidance on the use of economic claims, it is important to understand that the FDA does issue warning letters to pharmaceutical manufacturers who make false or misleading economic claims.[9]

This information may provide valuable insight into the current attitudes of the FDA and may serve as the basis for the future and final guidance on the subject.

Stewart et al.[9] conducted a qualitative study to examine the publicly available letters that were sent by the FDA to drug manufacturers for inappropriate promotional claims of specific medications. Of these 567 letters, 28 had false or misleading economic claims.[9] Of the 28 false or misleading claims, the most common violation, 14 (50 percent) contained, "unsupported comparative claim of effectiveness, safety, or interchangeability," contained "claims of cost savings when there are obvious additional costs that may affect cost savings," and 5 included "misleading price comparisons."[9]

These findings suggest that even without an official final guidance statement, the FDA has attempted to regulate material that contains economic claims. However, there is still uncertainty as to what constitutes an acceptable economic claim.

The Rofecoxib (Vioxx) Controversy: Refocusing on Safety

As of this writing, the FDA had not issued definitive guidance on the use of economic information concerning medications and because of recent events—may not for some time. With the 2004–2005 controversial events surrounding the FDA and the medication Vioxx, the ability of this U.S. agency to appropriately and impartially determine the safety of new healthcare technologies (its fundamental responsibility) is in question. The context of the controversy is hereto forth described.

In August 2004, Dr. David Graham, an official at the FDA, presented a research poster at the 20th International Conference on Pharmacoepidemiology and Therapeutic Risk Management in Bordeaux, France. The study examined the risk of acute myocardial infarction (i.e., heart attack) and sudden cardiac death among more than 1 million members of an HMO in California who received either a cyclooxygenase-2 inhibitor (the class of medications that includes Vioxx) or nonsteroidal anti-inflammatory (NSAID) medication (e.g., ibuprofen).[10] He and his colleagues found that a rofecoxib dose of greater than 25 mg per day was associated with a three-fold elevated risk of heart attack or sudden cardiac death as compared to NSAIDs.[10]

On September 30, 2004, rofecoxib was withdrawn from the market. On November 18, 2004, Graham stated that, "The FDA had ignored warnings that the pain pill was killing people by causing heart attacks and strokes."[11] On February 5, 2005, the *Lancet* published a study conducted by Graham and colleagues, which examined the side effects of rofecoxib among members of the California HMO. The investigation found that rofecoxib was associated with a 59 percent higher risk of coronary heart disease than celecoxib.

Interestingly, this publication was scheduled to be released on November 17, 2004, just 1 day before Graham was scheduled to testify before Congress on the inadequacies of the FDA procedures for monitoring the safety of medications. However, the publication was withdrawn on November 16.[12] Graham stated that:

> the FDA threatened him with "serious consequences" if he proceeded with publication of the study. The FDA did everything in its power to suppress [the findings] and keep them from public view.[12]

On February 17, 2005, Graham presented unpublished findings about the cardiovascular risks associated with a number of pain-relief medications at an expert panel meeting at the FDA. He stated that he was willing to present these study results because he had received a letter from the FDA acting commissioner saying he could do so without fear of retaliation.[13]

In an interesting twist that was unexpected by many in the policy arena, the FDA later recommended that the manufacturer reverse its withdrawal of Vioxx from the market. In doing so, the FDA acknowledged that the product had risks, but these risks could be addressed by improving the warning labels on the product.

In light of these events, the ability of the FDA to appropriately monitor the safety of healthcare technologies for the American public has come under much scrutiny. The issue of economic claims will in all likelihood take a second seat to safety issues.

Centers for Medicare and Medicaid Services

The Role of Economic Evaluation

CMS is responsible for the oversight of care for close to 50 million Americans as well as payment of over a billion dollars in healthcare interventions each and every day. With that much responsibility, one would expect that benefit coverage and payments are based on clear economic evaluations. Yet, this is not currently the case.

Although nothing in the federal statute explicitly prohibits Medicare from using cost-effectiveness analysis or any other type of economic evaluation to make decisions regarding coverage or reimbursement, CMS has been reluctant to do so. Perhaps this hesitation stems, in part, from the fact that American citizens and elected officials, have been unwilling to believe that healthcare resources are limited and do not understand that there are trade-offs between money and health.[4,14] To date, CMS has not published regulations or guidance documents that provide a definition of medical necessity or articulated the criteria that are applied to medical technologies in order to determine whether they are reasonable and necessary. This is a critical point, because coverage determinations are based on this undefined phrase. It has been suggested that the inability to execute a federal rule-making process aimed at defining the phrase reasonable and necessary is the result of society's discomfort with the inclusion of cost-effectiveness as one of the criteria.[15] A description of the process, though vague, appears in the *Federal Register* and can be found on the Medicare coverage Web site (www.cms.hhs.gov/coverage).

Allocating Healthcare Resources

Despite the limited role of economic evaluation in CMS decision making, significant progress has been made in making medical necessity decisions for the Medicare program.[5] There are three primary mechanisms through which CMS works to ensure healthcare resources are appropriately allocated for Medicare enrollees:

1. The use of evidence-based medicine to evaluate healthcare interventions
2. Requirement of a certificate of medical necessity for certain types of durable medical items
3. Healthcare quality initiatives

1. Use of Evidence-Based Medicine to Evaluate Healthcare Interventions
First, CMS evaluates clinical studies through a well-described framework of evidence-based medicine and posts decision memos on the Medicare coverage Web site. This site includes detailed explanations of what evidence was considered and how the coverage policy was derived.

2. Certificate of Medical Necessity
In addition, in some cases CMS places the responsibility for determining medical necessity into the hands of physicians through a certification process. A **Certificate of Medical Necessity** (CMN) is a form required by Medicare authorizing the use of certain durable medical items and equipment prescribed by a physician. This same system has been adapted by many other payors to assure appropriate coverage. The physician is also required to submit an updated CMN to CMS if there is a change in prescription and/or a change in the patient's condition.

3. Healthcare Quality Initiatives
When Medicare was first enacted in 1965, quality measurements could not be determined—so instead processes of care were measured in an attempt to ensure appropriate use of healthcare resources. Nowhere is this clearer than in the nursing home industry, which has long operated under heavy government regulation aimed at monitoring processes of care and achieving quality outcomes.

Furthermore, CMS requires healthcare providers to collect and monitor data on specific quality indicators (available at www.Medicare.gov). These requirements differ by type of provider, with nursing homes separate from hospitals, home care, and physicians. In addition to these quality measures, CMS has begun to publicize quality information on specific providers to consumers, in an effort to increase demand for providers that achieve the highest level of quality. The objective of this approach is to create an incentive for providers to achieve the quality goals that have been set forth by CMS. This concept has been suggested to be effective based on research showing that nursing home residents and their proxies respond to quality data by changing providers if necessary.[16]

Today, the Medicare payment policy is structured so as to align payments with provider performance. The **Medicare Payment Advisory Commission** (MedPAC) is required to consider a variety of measures because the direct relevance, availability, and quality of information in each potential indicator varies among providers.[17]

Nursing Home Quality Measurement

The Department of Health and Human Services (DHHS) has a national nursing home quality initiative to improve the quality of nursing home (NH) care. A critical part of this initiative is CMS's posting of quality indicators for every NH on 10 quality indicators.[18] These "report cards" are intended to be used by consumers to make informed decisions and motivate providers to improve their care. The CMS quality initiative is a major redirection to focus on clinical care needs of the frail elder instead of historically focusing on the process of care. This is the result of a shift toward the resident and away from the institution.

Hospital Quality Measures

CMS hospital quality measures come from information collected by hospitals that volunteer to provide data for public reporting. The information is intended to illustrate how quality of care can vary between hospitals. Currently, the quality information relates to the care given for patients with three serious medical conditions that are common in people with Medicare:

1. Myocardial infarction (i.e., heart attacks)
2. Congestive heart failure
3. Pneumonia

Hospital data are available from CMS through a partnership with the American Association of Retired Persons (AARP), American Federation of Labor (AFL/CIO), American Medical Association (AMA), Agency for Health Care Research and Quality (AHRQ), American Hospital Association (AHA), Association of American Medical Colleges (AAMC), Federation of American Hospitals (FAH), Joint Commission on Accreditation of Healthcare Organizations (JCAHO), and National Quality Forum (NQF). CMS first attempted to collect this information on a purely voluntary basis, but could not garner sufficient interest from hospitals. When voluntary participation failed, CMS tied submission of quality data to payments for services administered to Medicare patients. Today, hospitals that fail to submit data are not eligible for the payment increase applied to the payment, which can translate to as much as a 0.4 percent reduction in revenue for some facilities.[19]

Physician Quality Measures

Medicare payments for physician services are made on the basis of a fee schedule that has been in place since 1992. The Medicare fee schedule is intended to relate payments to the actual resources used in providing the healthcare services. The fee schedule assigns relative values to services that reflect physician work (i.e., time, skill, and intensity it takes to provide the service), practice expenses, and malpractice costs. These relative values are adjusted for geographic variations in costs.

Changes to this fee schedule (i.e, fee paid to physicians) are based on a Medicare law that specifies a formula for calculating the annual update in payments for physician services. The formula is controlled by limits placed on payment per service, but not on overall volume of services. As a result, the formula for calculating the annual change to the conversion factor responds to changes in volume. If the overall volume of services increases, the fee paid to physicians is lowered. In the last several years, the volume of services has increased; however, Congress allowed an increase rather than the required decrease in the fees paid to physicians.[20]

◼ Other Uses of Economic Evaluation

Although the CMS and FDA activities related to economic evaluation have been limited, one federal government program does use economic evaluation(s) as a means to guide policy decisions—the **Vaccines for Children program**. Since 1994, the Vaccines for Children program provides publicly purchased free vaccinations to all children who are eligible.[21] The vaccines and their associated dosing schedule(s) are recommended by the Advisory Committee on Immunization Practices (ACIP) and approved by the CDC.[21] Increasingly, national assessments of vaccinations include cost-effectiveness analysis (CEA).[22]

In 2000, the ACIP used information from a CEA to examine the then-new pneumococcal vaccine. According to the CEA included in the report on pneumonococcal disease in healthy children, vaccination is associated with a net savings if the vaccine costs less than $46 or $18 per dose, for the societal and healthcare payer perspectives, respectively.[23] The estimate for the societal net savings is more than twice that for the healthcare payer net savings because more than half of the estimated savings associated with the vaccine are from decreased workplace absenteeism by parents who care for ill children or secondary to pneumococcal disease (see Chapter 4).

The CDC accepted the ACIP recommendations for the vaccine, and the final price paid by the CDC for the vaccine was $44.25—almost the exact estimated cost associated with net savings from the societal perspective just noted.[1] Interestingly, this may suggest that this federal organization values the savings associated with decreased time lost from work and decreased lost workplace productivity (see Chapter 4).

Conclusion

Currently, the use of economic evaluation by U.S. regulators is quite limited, though the reasons for this are not clear. Is it due to political or cultural issues, or a lack of knowledge about the various economic techniques? However, as the costs associated with health care continue to rise and the available resources become increasingly limited, it seems inevitable that regulators will have to perform or at least use economic evaluations as a means to make informed decisions.

Due to current controversies within the FDA and the need to refocus the agency on ensuring the safety of new healthcare technologies, it is anticipated that it will be some time before the FDA issues a final guidance on the use of economic information on medications to healthcare practitioners. We have seen many times throughout the history of the FDA that the impetus for policy change and reform was an unfortunate national crisis. In moving forward, we are hopeful that regulators will prioritize activities involving economic evaluation as a tool to inform the trade-offs that will have to be made in order for the U.S. healthcare system to survive in the face of continued increases in the costs of technologies and the number of Americans receiving care.

Case Study

Streptococcus pneumoniae is the leading bacterial cause of meningitis, sepsis, pneumonia, and otitis media among U.S. children.[23] With the increased emergence of drug-resistant pneumococci, there is a need for preventive therapies that are effective. Unfortunately, some infants and young children do not respond well to the pneumococcal polysaccharide vaccine. A new vaccine that was approved by the FDA in February 2000, pneumococcal conjugate vaccine, was designed for use in such children and may further help to prevent the occurrence of pneumococcal disease.[23]

Suppose you are the medical director of a large managed care organization in the United States. You would like to determine if it is cost-effective for you to provide this new vaccine to your members. You would like to determine the projected health benefits, costs, and cost-effectiveness of routine pneumococcal conjugate vaccination of healthy infants in your managed care organization.

Consider the following questions:

1. What are the health benefits of the vaccine? To whom?
2. Do these benefits differ based on your study perspective (e.g., managed care versus society)?
3. What costs are associated with the vaccine and the disease?

4. Given your perspective as a medical director, justify why you would include and/or exclude certain identified costs in your estimations associated with the vaccine and the disease?
5. What data sources would you use to collect and measure the costs associated with the vaccine?
6. How would each of the identified costs be valued?
7. What type of economic evaluation would you use? Justify both the outcome selected and the methodology selected.

Study/Discussion Questions

1. What is the current role and use of economic evaluation in the CMS?
2. What are some of the various areas of healthcare services in which the CMS has enacted quality indicators?
3. What is the current role and use of economic evaluation in the U.S. Food and Drug Administration?
4. How has the CDC used economic evaluation?
5. What legislation allowed for the dissemination of health economic information of healthcare interventions to healthcare organizations?
6. What has/have been the impetus for much of the policy change and reform of the FDA in the 20th century?
7. What do you see as the future role of economic information and evaluation(s) by U.S. regulators?

Suggested Readings/Web Sites

Centers for Medicare and Medicaid Services. Medicare Coverage Homepage. Available at: www.cms.hhs.gov/coverage/.
Medicare: The Official U.S. Government Site for People with Medicare. Available at: www.medicare.gov.
Sinclair U. *The Jungle*. 1906. Available at: sinclair.thefreelibrary.com/Jungle.

References

1. Ruchlin HS, Dasbach EJ, Heyse JF. New directions in pharmacoeconomic research: The next step. *Drug Inf J*. 2002;36:909–917.
2. Swann JP. Food and Drug Administration. Kurian GT, ed. In: *A Historical Guide to the U.S. Government*. New York: Oxford University Press; 1998.
3. Higby GJ. The continuing evolution of American pharmacy practice. *J Am Pharm Assoc (Wash)*. 2002;42(1):12–15.

4. Neumann PJ. Why don't Americans use cost-effectiveness analysis? *Am J Manag Care.* 2004;10(5):308–312.

5. Tunis SR, Kang J. Improvements in medicare coverage of new technology. *Health Aff (Millwood).* 2001;20(5):83–85.

6. Merrill RA. Modernizing the FDA: An incremental revolution. *Health Aff (Millwood).* 1999;18(2):96–111.

7. Schwartz J. Another shot at FDA "Modernization"; bill to revamp food and drug agency draws less controversy than predecessor. *The Washington Post.* (1997, July 22): A13.

8. Kessler D. Statement by David A. Kessler Before the Committee on Labor and Human Resources (February 21, 1996). Available at: www.fda.gov/ola/1996/nktest.html. Accessed February 15, 2005.

9. Stewart KA, Neumann PJ. FDA actions against misleading or unsubstantiated economic and quality-of-life promotional claims: an analysis of warning letters and notices of violation. *Value Health.* 2002;5(5):389–396.

10. Matteson EL, Cush JJ, Kavanaugh A. (Hotline Editors) Cardiovascular Complications Related to COX-2 Inhibitors. April 5, 2002. Available at: www.rheumatology.org/publications/hotline/0904chfvioxx.asp. Accessed February 17, 2005.

11. Forbes. Face of the Year. December 13, 2004. Available at: www.forbes.com/sciencesandmedicine/2004/12/13/cx_mh_1213faceoftheyear.html. Accessed February 17, 2005.

12. Graham DJ, Campen D, Hui R, et al. Risk of acute myocardial infarction and sudden cardiac death in patients treated with cyclo-oxygenase 2 selective and non-selective non-steroidal anti-inflammatory drugs: Nested case-control study. *Lancet.* 2005;365(9458):475–478.

13. Globe Wire Services. February 17, 2005. FDA Clears Graham to Present Findings. Available at www.boston.com/yourlife/health/diseases/articles/2005/02/17/fda_clears_graham_to_present_findings?mode=PF. Accessed February 17, 2005.

14. Eddy DM. Clinical decision making: From theory to practice. Cost-effectiveness analysis. A conversation with my father. *JAMA.* 1992;267(12):1669–1675.

15. Tunis SR. Economic analysis in healthcare decisions. *Am J Manag Care.* 2004;10(5): 301–304.

16. Hirth RA, Banaszak-Holl JC, Fries BE, Turenne MN. Does quality influence consumer choice of nursing homes? Evidence from nursing home to nursing home transfers. *Inquiry.* 2003;40(4):343–361.

17. Tilson S, Chaikind H, O'Sullivan J, et al. CRS Report for Congress RL30526: Medicare Payment Policy. (updated February 23, 2005). Available at: www.law.umaryland.edu/marshall/crsreports/crsdocuments/RL3052602232005.pdf. Accessed March 1, 2005.

18. Nursing Home Compare. Medicare: The official U.S. government site for people with Medicare web site. July 2002. Available at: www.medicare.gov/NHCCompare/home.asp. Accessed February 15, 2005.

19. Centers for Medicare and Medicaid Services. Reporting Hospital Quality Data for Annual Payment Update. Fact Sheet. November 2004. Available at: www.cms.hhs.gov/quality/hospital/FactSheetAP.pdf. Accessed August 3, 2005.

20. O'Sullivan, J. CRS Report for Congress RL31199: Medicare Payments to Physicians. (Updated December 6, 2004). Available at: www.boozman.house.gov/UploadedFiles/MEDICARE%20-%20Physician%20Payments.pdf. Accessed February 15, 2005.

21. Centers for Disease Control and Prevention. Vaccines for Children Program: What Is the Public Health Issue? January 2004. Available at: www.cdc.gov/programs/immun11.htm. Accessed February 15, 2005.

22. Black S, Lieu TA, Ray GT, Capra A, Shinefield HR. Assessing costs and cost effectiveness of pneumococcal disease and vaccination within Kaiser Permanente. *Vaccine*. 2000;19(1):S83–S86.

23. Lieu TA, Ray GT, Black SB, et al. Projected cost-effectiveness of pneumococcal conjugate vaccination of healthy infants and young children. *JAMA*. 2000;283(11):1460–1468.

Chapter 9

THE FUTURE OF ECONOMIC EVALUATION WITHIN THE UNITED STATES

Jeffrey Clough
Al Crawford, PhD, MBA, MSIS
David B. Nash, MD, MBA

Overview

Economic evaluation is an important tool to determine the value of healthcare interventions. This chapter describes current initiatives related to the application of economic evaluation in U.S. healthcare decision making. Factors that influence the use of economic evaluation will be identified and discussed. A comparative analysis of international experience with economic evaluation will provide lessons on how to improve economic evaluation methods and promote their use in the United States.

Learning Objectives

1. To understand the forces driving the practice of economic evaluation in the U.S. healthcare system
2. To be able to understand international experiences with economic evaluation

3. To identify issues that are integral to the future success of economic evaluation in the United States.

Keywords

Canadian Coordination Office for Health Technology Assessment
Leapfrog Group
National Institute for Clinical Effectiveness
Patented Medicine Prices Review Board
Pharmaceutical Benefits Advisory Committee
Pharamceutical Benefits Group

Introduction

The U.S. healthcare system provides services that are vital to the health of the U.S. public. However, this system has finite resources to provide these services and so it is imperative that resources be allocated in a way that maximizes the public's health. As has been demonstrated throughout this book, economic evaluation is a tool for weighing the costs of healthcare interventions in relation to clinical, economic, or humanistic effects. As will be discussed in this chapter, the current decade may prove to be a crucial time for advances in the science and practice of economic evaluation.

In order to predict the future of economic evaluation in the United States, one must understand the current system. We begin by describing current initiatives to utilize economic evaluation in healthcare decision making. Next, we identify factors driving demand for this tool. Then, a comparative analysis of international experience with economic evaluation provides lessons to facilitate application of economic evaluation in the United States. We conclude with some important considerations for conducting economic evaluation in the future.

The Current Use of Economic Evaluation in the United States

Several healthcare organizations in the United States are beginning to utilize economic evaluation. As discussed in Chapter 8, the Centers for Medicare and Medicaid Services (CMS) is the largest healthcare payer in the nation. The pilot pay-for-performance projects mandated by the Medicare Modernization Act (MMA) of 2003 are CMS initiatives designed to specify and guarantee improved health outcomes. Another national organization making headway in this field is the Academy of Managed Care Pharmacy (AMCP), which provides drug dossiers incorporating economic evaluations of pharmaceuticals.[2] These dossiers may help pharmaceutical formulary managers select drugs that produce the best health outcomes for patients, given available budgets (see Chapter 7).

In addition, a number of U.S. universities and independent organizations have developed strategies for providing scientifically rigorous and objective economic evaluations. These include HAYES, Inc., of Lansdale, Pennsylvania; ECRI of Plymouth Meeting, Pennsylvania; and Abt Associates, Inc., of Cambridge, Massachusetts.[3,4,5] There have also been proposals for public support to develop additional independent organizations. One such proposal is the expansion of the Centers for Education and Research on Therapeutics (CERTs). There are currently four such centers, supported by the U.S. Agency for Healthcare Research and Quality (AHRQ), that perform research on issues such as prescribing errors, adverse reactions, and real-market based outcomes. Future CERT programs may include economic evaluation.[6] One prominent health economist, Dr. Uwe Reinhardt, has gone so far as to call for an independent pharmacoeconomics research institute.[7] Such an organization would require support by professional organizations to foster credibility in its work.

Despite the examples described, there is currently little utilization of economic evaluation in the U.S. healthcare system. To understand why this paucity of economic evaluation exists, one must look at the structure of the U.S. healthcare system. As Donald Berwick, CEO of the Institute for Healthcare Improvement, stated: "Every system is perfectly designed to produce exactly the results that it gets."[8] Unlike most market-driven industries, the U.S. healthcare industry lacks the necessary components to create demand for value (i.e., better health outcomes at a lower cost). These components include benchmarking, standardization, and continuous measurement and improvement of healthcare services. The U.S. healthcare system has been described as a "zero-sum game" in which the system is designed to divide value rather than create it; in this system, payers and providers compete only to shift costs and evade accountability for the quality or efficiency of the care they provide.[9] Economic evaluation will emerge as a significant tool for improving healthcare quality and value only when the system rewards value instead of cost reduction.

How Can U.S. Decision Makers Be Motivated to Adopt Economic Evaluation?

Many forces are driving the demand for greater healthcare value in the United States. Although it is hard to predict change in a healthcare system as complex as the United States, a useful framework for understanding and predicting such change, developed by David Gustafson and associates, includes four drivers (Figure 9-1):

1. Tension for change
2. Existence of a superior alternative
3. Skills and self-efficacy for change
4. Public support.[10]

Each of these drivers is discussed below.

Figure 9-1 Drivers of Change That Will Stimulate U.S. Adoption of Economic Evaluation

1. Tension for change	Rising healthcare costs; variations in healthcare quality
2. Superior alternative	Economic evaluations can reduce costs and increase quality
3. Skills and self-efficacy	Global efforts to advance science of economic evaluation
4. Public support	Employer efforts (Leapfrog Group); recognition of costs by patients; MMA pay-for-performance projects

Source: Gustafson, et al., 1992.

Organizational Driver 1: Tension for Change

In the current environment of rising U.S. health expenditures, limited resources, and new technologies, the need for economic evaluation is increasing. Healthcare expenditures consumed 15.3 percent of the U.S. Gross Domestic Product (GDP), and are projected to nearly 18.7 percent of the GDP by 2014.[11] This tension affects all stakeholders in the United States. Health plans struggle to contain costs without compromising quality of care. In turn, providers often resent and distrust restrictions imposed by health plans. The division between these two key stakeholders results in large part from the lack of reliable information about the clinical effectiveness and cost-effectiveness of therapies.

In response to increased expenditures, health plans raise premiums—which negatively impacts patients and payers. Employers and insurers then seek relief from escalating costs by shifting costs to employees through increased copayments, deductibles, premiums, or reduced covered services. In turn, employees with less coverage may forego expensive but necessary treatment, which generates more costs as their health conditions worsen.

As a major payor for healthcare services in the United States, government (both at the federal and state levels) is also significantly affected by the escalating healthcare costs. Some analysts predict that the Medicare trust fund will be exhausted as early as 2019.[12] Although CMS has traditionally been a passive payer, it is expected to assume a more active role in coverage decisions and to start measuring and managing the outcomes of the services for which it reimburses.

Another important source of tension is the realization by patients that there is a wide gap between what they expect from the healthcare system and what it actually delivers. Highly publicized reports, such as an Institute of Medicine (IOM) report, which stated that medical errors are responsible for up to 100,000 deaths annually, highlight significant variations in outcomes among providers.[13] Additionally, comparisons of the United States to other developed countries suggest that the greater per capita healthcare expenditures may not effectively improve the health of the population.[14] These factors are leading patients to demand both transparency of healthcare information and accountability for the costs and outcomes of health care, rather than passively accepting providers' assurances. To the degree that patients demand information and select providers based on outcomes, providers will compete to improve healthcare outcomes and value.

Organizational Driver 2: Superior Alternative

Using an economic evaluation to aid decisions about healthcare interventions should be superior to ignoring economic information. Industries that are accountable for the quality and cost of their products have seen substantial quality improvements and cost reductions through competition. Ideally, incorporating economic evaluation in the healthcare decision-making process can both control costs and produce the best possible quality of care. The Midwest Business Group on Health (MBGH) estimated that poor quality costs the United States up to $600 billion, in direct and indirect costs, annually.[15] Economic evaluation, used appropriately, is the best tool available for comparing the costs and outcomes of different treatment options.

Organizational Driver 3: Skills and Self-Efficiency

One of the most important factors promoting the use of economic evaluation in health care is the burgeoning research in this field. The *Gold Book* helped to improve and standardize the techniques of cost-effectiveness analysis.[16] Many academic institutions have developed programs in health economics or pharmacoeconomics. The growing utilization and sophistication of economic evaluation internationally and the global integration of this science by organizations such as the International Society for Pharmacoeconomics and Outcomes Research (ISPOR) also enhance the scientific validity and legitimacy of such studies. The experience of numerous governments provides real-life examples of problems encountered when performing economic evaluations. Though the science of economic evaluation in health care is relatively young, the field is advancing and should continue to progress in the future.

Organizational Driver 4: Social Support

Public support is a critical component of any major policy change in a democratic society. Although successful public health interventions are based on science, there is an important political component as well. For instance, public health efforts in the 20th century virtually eliminated diphtheria in the United States. However, this achievement was not accomplished solely by scientific discoveries of the nature of the disease, but also by heightened public awareness and innovative programs.[17]

Historically, there has been very little support in the United States for allocating healthcare services based on economic considerations. Consequently, the government has been reluctant to rely on economic evaluation in decisions to cover health services. For instance, the Food and Drug Administration (FDA) does not require cost-effectiveness data to be submitted in support of a new drug. Additionally, the U.S. Preventive Services Task Force (USPSTF) includes cost-effectiveness studies when analyzing preventive services, but it does not explicitly rank these services based on these data.[18]

The private sector may have little incentive to use formal economic evaluation because quality health outcomes are typically not rewarded in the United States. Additionally, there may be suspicion that this sector uses economic evaluation only to increase profits, rather than to provide better patient outcomes. Health plans have faced litigation over services they consider unnecessary, and it is unclear whether formal economic evaluation will help them defend against such litigation.[19] Healthcare policymakers and decision makers face a major challenge in creating support for incorporating value determinations in healthcare policies and decisions.

However, there is some hope that the public will eventually recognize the need for weighing the outcomes and costs of health care. This recognition will be stimulated by the shifting of healthcare costs from payers to patients. Historically, patients were sheltered from healthcare expenses because insurance plans paid providers directly and patients had relatively small copayments, deductibles, and premiums. In an effort to control costs, many payers are now requiring patients to contribute a greater share of their healthcare costs. This shift may make patients more cognizant of what resources they are consuming and more discriminating in terms of what services they are willing to pay for. It is likely that this trend will continue and more patients will demand to know the actual benefits of the health care they are purchasing.

There has also been a growing demand by employers for accountability in health care. One prominent example is the **Leapfrog Group**, a consortium of large employers that rate providers on measures such as utilization of electronic patient records and of intensivists in intensive care units.[20] Since employers purchase most privately funded health care, their increasing demand for value will influence the entire healthcare system. One major challenge will be to align the incentives of employers with those of employees. If employers do not communicate the value of selected health plans to employees, then only employers will have the incentive to reduce costs, not employees themselves. Thus, better communication between these two stakeholders is needed to reward employers who select better providers for their employees.

Finally, there is evidence that even public payers support selectively purchasing healthcare services based on value. Passage of the Medicare Modernization Act (MMA) was the largest expansion of public healthcare spending in the United States since the inception of the Medicare and Medicaid programs in 1965. MMA requires development of two pay-for-performance pilot projects, which will require that participating providers both reduce costs and improve quality to receive full payment.[21] If successful, these projects will demonstrate that CMS can assume a more active role in demanding better outcomes.

Clearly there is a need to measure the effects and costs of health care so that the system can best accomplish its purpose, which is to improve the health of the public. Economic evaluation is the best tool available to meet this need, but variation in the quality and results of evaluations performed in recent years has stifled adoption. Many stakeholders have expressed frustration that decisions made using economic data are often inconsistent and influenced by subjective factors. Fortunately, the international community is making efforts to improve the scientific rigor and effective use of economic evaluations in health care. Such initiatives will provide many lessons to help advance this field within the United States and abroad.

What Can be Learned from International Experience?

Despite limited use of economic evaluation in the United States, there is an international movement to advance the science. Most developed nations currently have legislation, public policies, and organizations mandating use of economic evaluation in at least one sector of the healthcare industry, most often the pharmaceutical sector. In this age of increasing globalization, it is possible to learn from the successes and failures of programs in other nations. Communication via the Internet and international organizations such as ISPOR promote the global dissemination and integration of economic information. As the scientific merit of economic evaluations and the ability to effectively apply results increases internationally, the capacity for all nations to maximize their populations' health will theoretically increase.

This section will describe three countries' approaches to economic evaluation, in the United Kingdom, Canada, and Australia. A summary of these approaches is provided in Table 9-1. The strengths and limitations of these different approaches will be highlighted, and lessons will be extracted that may be applicable to the U.S. healthcare system. The discussion will illustrate how international experiences in this field can provide valuable information, even though the U.S. healthcare system differs significantly from other countries.

The United Kingdom Experience

Economic evaluation in the United Kingdom usually occurs within a process formally known as Health Technology Assessment (HTA). HTA in the United Kingdom involves the assessment not only of pharmaceuticals and devices, but also procedures and organizational and support systems.[22] Economic evaluation is the most prominent component of HTA, but other components include analyses of ethical and social consequences.[22] The HTA process has been employed since the early 1990s in the United Kingdom's National Health Service (NHS). The establishment of the **National Institute for Clinical Excellence** (NICE) in 1999 created a formal distinction between *assessments* and *appraisals* of health technologies. Assessments are objective evaluations of technologies, whereas appraisals are subjective decisions about whether to use the technologies. Assessments may be con-

Table 9-1 Summary of International Organizations Conducting Economic Evaluations

International Organizations Conducting Economic Evaluations	Description	Strengths*	Limitations
NICE (United Kingdom)	Appraises health technologies; decisions must be funded by NHS	Decision making solicits opinions from all stakeholders	Economic evaluations only include NHS perspective; focus on pharmaceuticals
PMPRB (Canada)	Economic evaluations justify regulating pharmaceutical prices	Has reduced pharmaceutical costs	May limit research and development of new pharmaceuticals
CCOHTA (Canada)	Provides objective economic evaluations for decision makers	Evaluations are conducted from societal perspective	Decision makers may alter the evaluations to their needs
PBAC (Australia)	Evaluates outpatient pharmaceuticals to be subsidized for all Australians	Includes perspective of entire health budget; relatively consistent in decisions	Evaluations of variable quality; may not capture benefits outside health department
Drug and Therapeutic Committees (Australia)	Evaluates inpatient therapies to be used in individual institution	Can conduct evaluations customized to individual population	Very little oversight of quality or use of evaluations

*Strengths and limitations are based on the authors' evaluation.

ducted by several organizations, but NICE makes the final appraisal decisions for the technologies that it considers. Before the establishment of NICE, decisions about which technologies to fund were made by a variety of organizations at the national or local level. In contrast, NICE is a centralized group. The NHS is required by law to fund its operation and to guarantee that its recommendations are available throughout the United Kingdom. NICE applies explicit criteria for selecting technologies to appraise, and a standard format for appraisal (Figure 9-2). The NICE panel allows input from patient groups, clinical experts, and manufacturers. After NICE issues a recommendation as to whether to fund a healthcare technology, manufacturers, professionals, and other parties have the opportunity to appeal the decision if they believe it be incorrect.

Although the NICE system is still evolving, there is a growing body of expert commentary on its strengths and weaknesses. Compared to HTA systems in other countries, NICE has more explicit criteria and procedures for technology review. This is helpful to manufacturers as they prepare to introduce a new product.[21] Additionally, the process is visible and publicly accessible and allows input from a wide variety of stakeholders. In particular, NICE has been commended for most effectively incorporating the perspective of patient advocates, compared to other programs.[23] This helps prevent political tensions that might arise if decisions were made privately or if one or more parties were not allowed to participate fully. Weatherly et al. surveyed sources of information used by health improvement programs, which are programs used by local health authorities to improve health and health care, and found that NICE recommendations are considered the best source of advice on economic considerations.[24]

Figure 9-2 Criteria for Selecting Technologies for Appraisal by NICE

The Department of Health and the National Assembly for Wales will select technologies for appraisal based on the following criteria:

- Is the technology likely to result in a significant health benefit, taken across the NHS as a whole, if given to all patients for whom it is indicated?
- Is the technology likely to result in a significant impact on other health-related government policies (e.g., reduction in health inequalities)?
- Is the technology likely to have a significant impact on NHS resources (financial or other) if given to all patients for whom it is indicated?
- Is the Institute likely to be able to add value by issuing national guidance? For instance, in the absence of such guidance, is there likely to be significant controversy over the interpretation or significance of the available evidence on clinical and cost-effectiveness?

Note: These criteria are set and applied jointly by the (English) Department of Health and the National Assembly of Wales.

Source: Adapted from Stevens A and Milne R. Health Technology Assessment in England and Wales. *International Journal of Technology Assessment in Health Care,* 20:1(2004),11–24. Reprinted with permission of Cambridge University Press.

However, there have been important criticisms of the NICE process. Political scientists have commented that allowing lobbying to influence the appraisal process may harm NICE's image of objectivity.[25] Critics also argue that NICE is reluctant to make negative recommendations for political reasons.[26] Also, given that NICE's economic evaluations must take the perspective of the NHS, costs and benefits for other sectors or levels of government, or society at large, are not necessarily included.[27]

Another major criticism concerns the focus of NICE appraisals. From its establishment in 1999 until January 2002, two thirds of NICE appraisals addressed pharmaceuticals, even though this sector accounts for only 10 to 15 percent of total healthcare costs.[27] Also, the need to supply economic data to obtain a positive NICE recommendation may require expensive trials, which increases development costs, and ultimately the prices, of new drugs.[21] In contrast, there have been few economic evaluations of nonpharmaceutical products or services that could improve health outcomes, such as medical procedures or public health interventions.[28] Finally, because NICE only reviews a small percentage of emerging technologies and positive recommendations must be funded, it is possible that less cost-effective technologies are funded simply because they were selected for appraisal while more cost-effective technologies were simply not appraised.

What Can We Learn from the United Kingdom?
Although the U.S. healthcare system is more complex than the U.K. system (e.g., with multiple payers rather than a single payer) it is still possible to draw lessons from the NICE experience. NICE has advantages in that the U.K. system is centralized and recommendations are universally implemented. An analogous organization performing economic evaluation in the United States would not have comparable power given the multipayer system. However, economic evaluation conducted by a national organization, viewed as representing the interests of society, might have considerable credibility. Thus, even though such an organization's recommendations might not be mandated, they might be widely adopted by providers and payers. For such an organization to be effective, it would need input from all stakeholders, including patients, providers, and manufacturers, to develop and facilitate acceptance of its recommendations. It would also need to disclose publicly its methods, data, and results—so that other evaluators might replicate and validate its findings.

NICE's public stance is that it does not ration health care. Far from being merely a matter of semantics, this policy is very pertinent to the United States. The Oregon Department of Human Services lost public support in the 1990s because the word "rationing" was used to describe its program (see Chapter 1). Given their mission to select the most cost-effective healthcare technologies, NICE and other HTA groups must sometimes restrict access to clinically effective technologies that are too costly to justify their consumption of limited resources. Critics argue that NICE's refusal to call this "rationing" in order to protect its image obfuscates its purpose and weakens its position.[26] Any U.S. organization conducting economic evaluation of healthcare services may be similarly tempted to avoid politically sensitive language. However, if NICE ultimately proves unsuccessful at reducing use of ineffective technologies, future U.S. organizations might consider taking a stronger position against political pressure.

The Canadian Experience

The **Patented Medicine Prices Review Board** (PMPRB), founded in 1987, is an independent body that performs annual reviews of the prices of all Canadian patented medications. Given that the federal payer, Health Canada, does not cover pharmaceuticals used outside of the hospital, the PMPRB is an important mechanism to control excessive drug prices. The PMPRB review process provides explicit criteria for evaluating the appropriateness of patented medication prices, including analyzing cost-effectiveness, making cross-national price comparisons, and considering manufacturers' profit margins. For breakthrough drugs, manufacturers must submit relevant data, including findings published in scientific journals. If the price of a medication is judged to be excessive, the PMPRB may lower the price or fine the manufacturer.[29] The PMPRB only has jurisdiction over the price that the manufacturer charges wholesalers, hospitals, or pharmacies and cannot control prices that these intermediaries charge consumers.

The PMPRB uses economic evaluation to inform and justify direct price controls. These controls have had some success in controlling pharmaceutical spending in Canada. Between 1987 and 1999, the ratio of Canadian drug prices to median prices of the same drugs in seven comparable Organisation for Economic Co-operation and Development (OECD) countries fell from 1.23 to 0.90; additionally, 97 percent of breakthrough drugs in Canada were priced below the median prices in the seven comparable OECD countries in 1999, compared to only 75 percent in 1990.[30]

However, PMPRB price controls have been criticized for diminishing pharmaceutical firms' investment in research and development. Additionally, critics have argued that some drugs have not been introduced in Canada because of price controls (e.g., Ambien, Capozide, Orelox, and Lorabid). Others have pointed out that focusing on prices may not be the best way to control drug costs, advocating, instead, for a broader approach incorporating physicians' prescribing patterns, utilization, and demographic and other patient attributes.

The other key Canadian organization is the **Canadian Coordinating Office for Health Technology Assessment** (CCOHTA), an independent, nonprofit organization that has performed economic evaluations since 1989. CCOHTA's goal is to provide information to decision makers regarding the cost-effectiveness of health technologies. Given that decisions about which technologies to fund are typically made at the provincial level, the CCOHTA board of directors represents the ministries of health of each province and territory. Pharmacy directors in government, hospitals, and advisory committees to Health Canada use CCOHTA reports. Although the CCOHTA does not make the final decision to fund technologies, it does issue guidelines for economic evaluations of them.[31]

The CCOHTA differs from the NICE model in that assessment is centralized but appraisal is decentralized. This separation is beneficial in that it maintains the perceived objectivity and credibility of CCOHTA reports. In addition, decision makers can reanalyze the data and adapt the findings to the requirements of their respective populations. This decentralization of decision making allows for variation in adoption of technologies; however, there is concern that such variation may not serve the needs of these various populations.

Another feature of the Canadian model is that decision makers may complete an economic evaluation from their own perspective, even though CCOHTA's guidelines recommend use of the societal perspective. In particular, decisions about which drugs to include on a formulary are often constrained by a fixed budget and thus focus only on minimizing costs within that budget. Accordingly, a formulary committee with a constrained budget might reject an expensive drug that increases hospital costs, even though its approval and widespread utilization would be valuable to an integrated organization of providers and patients, and to society as a whole.

What Can We Learn from Canada?
Organizational designs similar to those of the PMPRB and CCOHTA may be more feasible in the United States than the NICE design, because they do not rely on national decision making. Although legislation creating an institution similar to the PMPRB would probably meet with strong resistance from the pharmaceutical lobby in this country, some experts predict that governmental price controls for pharmaceuticals will eventually emerge.[32] With passage of the MMA in 2003, CMS may indeed take the initiative to limit reimbursement for some of the drugs it covers.

If this occurs, it will be interesting to see how prices negotiated or set by CMS extend to other public and private payers. Pharmaceutical firms could not afford to forego the enormous and dominant U.S. market, and most other national markets have at least some price controls. As shown in Canada, price controls can be effective in lowering prices. However, there is still debate about whether this limits investment in research and development. Perhaps it would be more prudent for the United States to take a broader perspective in controlling expenditures on pharmaceuticals by targeting other factors such as ineffective prescribing practices by physicians and inappropriate utilization by patients.

An independent organization similar to the CCOHTA could be developed in the United States. Since the U.S. healthcare system has many payers, public and private, an independent organization could employ standardized methods and perform objective, credible evaluations. It would then be the responsibility of providers and health plans to decide which technologies are most appropriate for their constituencies, taking into account the characteristics, values, and financial resources of the patient populations they serve.

A major issue in the United States, as occurred in Canada, is how to discourage evaluators from employing only their own perspective rather than a societal perspective. One method to counteract this tendency would be to require decisions to be made at the broadest possible level. Additionally, the patient perspective should be considered by including patient advocates in decision making. Another approach would be to guarantee that information about health outcomes is universally available; in a truly competitive environment, this would align the perspectives of patients, payers, and providers.

The Australian Experience

Australia has several organizations that incorporate economic evaluations into healthcare assessment. Most importantly, the **Pharmaceutical Benefits Advisory Committee** (PBAC) conducts economic evaluations of pharmaceuticals. These evaluations are usually based on analyses submitted by pharmaceutical companies according to standard guidelines. New drugs meeting safety and efficacy requirements may be submitted to the PBAC for consideration to be covered by the **Pharmaceutical Benefits Scheme** (PBS).

The PBS provides subsidies for outpatient drugs on its registry for all Australian citizens. The PBAC must recommend new drugs that are cost-effective for possible inclusion in the PBS and has the options of (1) recommending covering the drug with no restrictions, (2) covering the drug at a lower price, (3) covering the drug for restricted populations, or (4) not covering the drug at all. Ultimately, the Minister of Health and Aging negotiates the price to be paid by the PBS. These negotiations rely primarily on analyses by the PBAC, but include other factors such as international prices for the drug, potential misuse of the drug, and manufacturers' profits.

PBAC evaluations are usually conducted from the government perspective although patient copayments are often considered as well. Comparators for the drug being evaluated are, in order of priority, the most frequently used analogue, a different drug, or nondrug medical management for the same indication. Such evaluations have had mixed results. George and associates found a significant correlation between the incremental cost-effectiveness ratio (ICER) and inclusion decisions by the PBS.[33] However, studies have found variation in the quality of PBAC analyses. For example, a study reported that two thirds of economic evaluations used by the PBAC had major problems, including lack of good data, poor assumptions in modeling, and even calculation errors.[34] Moreover, Australia's efforts have had limited success in slowing the growth of total drug expenditures, which have increased as rapidly as those of other OECD countries.[35] However, it is not clear whether this increase in drug spending has been accompanied by decreases in other forms of healthcare spending.

In addition to the PBAC-PBS system, nearly all hospitals have a drug and therapeutic committees (DTCs) responsible for education and policy, mostly regarding medications. The committees consist mostly of clinicians, although other stakeholders may be involved.[36] Weekes and Brooks found that most DTCs use guidelines, prescribing restrictions, or pharmacist monitoring to implement their policies.[36] Although DTCs are not strictly regulated, Weekes and Brooks developed a set of indicators to evaluate their work.[36] However, there is little information regarding the use, scientific rigor, and consistency of economic evaluations by DTCs.

What Can We Learn from Australia?
Australia's PBAC-PBS system is similar to Canada's PMPRB system in that cost-effectiveness evaluations are used to inform and justify pharmaceutical price controls. One major distinction of Australia's system is that drug costs are set and reimbursed by the same organization. This may be a useful model for the CMS to emulate for the Medicare prescription drug benefit. As in the Australian system, Medicare benefits will include both inpatient and outpatient medical and pharmacy benefits. As currently structured, these different types of coverage are "silos"; that is, separately funded services that allow limited opportunities for comprehensive management. Ideally, the costs and benefits of all healthcare services covered by Medicare and Medicaid should be integrated in comprehensive analyses of the cost-effectiveness of drugs. However, it remains to be seen how implementation of the MMA will affect these issues.

An additional limitation in the United States lies in the fact that Medicare covers only senior citizens. Even after the Medicare drug benefit is implemented, private payers covering employees and other nonsenior members will still have responsibility for formulary decisions and drug price negotiations. It is likely that problems with the effectiveness and quality of economic evaluations will persist, because decisions remain largely decentralized. An important issue will be how to measure and improve the quality of economic evaluations and subsequent decision making. Developing quality indicators for economic evaluation organizations analogous to those developed for Australia's DTCs may improve levels of standardization and quality across these decentralized organizations. Otherwise, it is likely that variations in the rationales, perspectives, and capabilities of organizations performing economic evaluation in the United States will produce variations in the quality of their analyses and decisions and in how well they reflect the needs and values of the U.S. population.

Issues in the Future Use of Economic Evaluation in the United States

Drawing on the lessons learned from other countries allows identification of important considerations related to the future use of economic evaluation in the United States. One of these lessons is to ensure that all appropriate interests are considered in any government-required evaluation of a drug or technology. Another lesson learned is that national bodies must promote the acceptance of the results of economic evaluation, particularly among physicians. Consideration of these issues provides a platform for predicting what types of programs may be used to conduct economic evaluation in the United States in the future.

Integration of Appropriate Interests into Economic Evaluation

The perspective of the evaluator can have a significant impact on the results of an evaluation. Additionally, the needs of the decision maker may influence whether and how the evaluation results are utilized. The NICE and PBAC-PBS systems incorporate the broadest perspective, namely that of the national healthcare system. However, their evaluations do not capture certain societal costs and benefits such as lost productivity and costs of care provided by patients' families. In these cases, even though there is a single payer (the national government) not all costs and benefits are captured if they do not specifically accrue to that institution.

In the Canadian system, analyses theoretically include all relevant institutions. However, there is no mechanism to prevent individual decision makers (i.e., provincial health plans and formularies) from adapting the evaluations based on their specific perspectives. Finally, Australian DTCs have virtually no oversight of the perspectives used in their evaluations.

This issue of perspective is certain to be even more complex in the United States, with its many independent payers, both private and public. Some relevant questions include: Who will fund and conduct the evaluations? Who will ultimately make the appraisal decisions? What mechanisms will assure that evaluations are conducted and utilized from acceptable perspectives?

If organizations are developed in the United States to conduct independent economic evaluations, will they employ a societal perspective, as recommended by ISPOR, to maximize their credibility and legitimacy? A major challenge will be preventing individual payers, such as health insurers and pharmacy benefit managers (PBMs), from conducting or adapting evaluations based only on their specific needs, such as cost minimization within their budget, without considering the effects on other institutions. One approach to this problem would be federal legislation to regulate the perspective to be used in economic evaluations, perhaps accompanied by compliance monitoring. However, such legislation would most likely be viewed as antithetical to the values of the American market economy, and, in any event, it would be difficult to enforce, because economic evaluations require many assumptions.

A second approach would be to align the incentives of decision makers with those of society. Specifically, if excellent health outcomes are among society's most important objectives, outcomes should be measured and publicized so that patients can choose healthcare providers that optimize outcomes. Competitive pressures to optimize outcomes might also induce providers to make strategic alliances to mitigate detrimental "silo" effects. For instance, a PBM might debate covering a costly drug that will both improve patients' health and reduce hospitalization costs. However, the PBM or payer might not be able to afford to put the drug on the formulary. A solution might be for the PBM to partner strategically with the health plan paying patients' hospitalization costs to share the savings and thus benefit both organizations, as well as the patients. This second approach will likely be favored over the first, because it is more consistent with the free-market values and preferences of American society.

It is important to recognize that evaluators will not be able to acquire sufficient funding to assess every medication, device, procedure, or preventive measure, and they will have to prioritize what they assess. Funding for these evaluations will have to be provided by parties with an interest in their results. If at any point, the expected value of the information obtained from an economic evaluation is less than the cost of the evaluation, conducting the evaluation becomes counterproductive and it will face resistance by patients and providers.

Credibility of Economic Evaluations

The acceptance of economic evaluation in the U.S. healthcare system will require acceptance of the idea that economic studies can maximize health outcomes—not just reduce costs. Although payers may understand the value of such evaluations, providers and patients often resist reliance on economic factors when making healthcare decisions. This resistance stems from the American belief that health care is a basic human right. Although it is widely recognized that there are insufficient resources to provide unlimited health care and that a lack of provider accountability produces suboptimal outcomes, providers and patients often mistrust and resent payers, who are perceived to ration care only to save money.

How Can Economic Evaluations Gain Credibility with Patients?
In the United States, patients have limited control over demand for healthcare,

because third parties such as employers or government are the direct purchasers. However, patients have a powerful influence through public opinion and the political system. Fear of public backlash has most likely been a major barrier to incorporating economic evaluations in the policies of organizations such as the U.S. Preventive Services Task Force (USPSTF), FDA, and CMS.

In the private sector, managed care organizations (MCOs) have been highly criticized for withholding care. Politicians and the media often portray MCOs as being profit hungry, so MCOs are wary about openly using economic evaluation. Although public support may continue to grow based on increasing awareness of escalating costs and variable quality, it will be important for MCOs that conduct economic evaluations to make it clear that their mission to provide the highest quality care for patients. This may best be demonstrated by sponsorship of evaluation activities by respected organizations, such as physician organizations and patient advocacy groups.

How Can Economic Evaluations Gain Credibility with Physicians?
Historically, physicians have been primarily responsible for allocating healthcare resources in the United States. They are influenced not only by the individual needs of their patients, but also by administrative regulations, restrictions, and incentives. Any attempt to implement cost-effective healthcare will likely fail without the endorsement and cooperation of physicians.

There is a large body of research describing the unnecessary variation in physician decisions and factors that may contribute to this variation.[37] Since the successful use of economic evaluations in health care will require compliance with a specified regimen, physicians must find ways to limit this variation. A good starting point is teaching skills that will help physicians understand and evaluate the impact of their decisions on the entire healthcare system.

Although the medical profession has been slow to train physicians to maximize health outcomes in a system-based manner, there are several promising initiatives in medical education. The Accreditation Council for Graduate Medical Education (ACGME) will soon require all residency programs to teach and assess residents in "systems-based practice" and "practice-based learning and improvement."[38] While not aimed at economic evaluation, these requirements will help the next generation of physicians to understand how their actions influence the broader healthcare system and also assess and improve the quality of their practices. Incorporation of public health into medical school curriculum will also help to mold physicians to have a societal perspective.

In addition to these skills, physicians will need to be able to understand and critique economic evaluations. Although this is not yet a component of traditional medical education, there are checklists available to aid physicians (see Chapter 2). Managers of healthcare organizations that make decisions based on economic evaluations must make sure that physicians understand the rationale behind these decisions and endorse them. If physicians' opinions are not adequately represented, their resentment may adversely affect the implementation of those decisions.

Conclusion

The U.S. healthcare system cannot afford to continue funding care without understanding the value of that care. Economic evaluation is a key tool for objectively measuring this value. Specifically, economic evaluation can provide information needed to redirect competitive forces in healthcare from an emphasis solely on reducing costs to one of creating better patient outcomes.

The combined efforts of the international economic evaluation community will be instrumental in stimulating its adoption in the United States. The globalization and democratization of information can benefit all parties. As the use of economic evaluation expands and improves, the sharing of techniques and information will raise the quality, accountability, and legitimacy of this emerging discipline. Physicians, patients, and payers must understand that economic evaluation is needed to help allocate scarce healthcare resources. Payors must seek to involve all parties in such decisions to ensure their efficacious implementation. The health of the public is ultimately linked, in large measure, to the decisions behind the allocation of healthcare resources. The tools of economic evaluation can facilitate an often complicated decision-making process.

Study/Discussion Questions

1. Why will the importance of economic evaluation continue to increase in the United States?
2. What lessons have been learned from other countries about the potential application of economic evaluation in the United States?
3. How might the practice of economic evaluation be stimulated in the United States?

Suggested Readings/Web Sites

Australia: Pharmaceutical Benefits Advisory Committee (PBAC). Available at: www.health.gov.au.internet/wcms/publishing.nsf/Content/health-pbs-general-listing-committee.htm.

Canada: Patented Medicine Prices Review Board (PMPRB). Available at: www.pmprb-cepmb.gc.ca.

Canadian Coordinating Office for Health Technology Assessment (CCOHTA). Available at: www.ccohta.ca.

International Journal of Technology Assessment in Health Care. Available at: journals.cambridge.org/bin/bladerunner?30REQEVENT=&REQAUTH=0&116000RE QSUB==&REQSTR1=THC.

United Kingdom: National Institute for Clinical Excellence (NICE). Available at: www.nice.org.uk.

References

1. Stevens A, Milne R. Health technology assessment in England and Wales. *Int J Technol Assess Health Care.* 2004;20(1)11–24.

2. Nash DB. The AMCP's drug dossier format. *P&T.* 2003;28(10):624.

3. Hayes, Inc. 2004. Available at: www.hayesinc.com. Accessed December 15, 2004.

4. ECRI. 2004. Available at: www.ecri.org. Accessed December 15, 2004.

5. Abt Associates, Inc. Available at: www.abtassociates.com/index.cfm2004. Accessed December 15, 2004.

6. Nash DB. CERTainly a great idea! *P&T.* 2001;26(6):285.

7. Reinhardt U. An information infrastructure for the pharmaceutical market. *Health Aff (Millwood).* 2004;23(1):107–112.

8. Phillips DF. New look reflects changing style of patient safety enhancement. *JAMA.* 1999;281(3):217–219.

9. Porter M, Teisberg E. Redefining competition in health care. *Harv Bus Rev.* 2004;82(6)65–76.

10. Gustafson D, Alemi F, Cats-Baril W. *Systems to Support Health Policy Analysis: Theory, Models and Uses.* Ann Arbor, MI: Health Administration Press; 1992.

11. Heffler S, Smith S, Keehan S, Borger C, Clemens MK, Truffer C. Trends: U.S. Health spending projections for 2004–2014. *Health Aff (Millwood).* 2005:w5.74–85. Available at: content.healthaffairs.org/cgi/reprint/hlthaff.w5.74v1. Accessed May 10, 2005.

12. Tieman J. Medicare Madness: Debate over the recently passed reform law is showing no sign of subsidising as wary providers brace for budget-busting backlash. *Mod Healthc.* 2004;34(13):4–5.

13. Institute of Medicine. *To Err Is Human: Building a Safer Health System.* Washington, DC: National Academy Press; 2000.

14. Hussey P, Anderson G, Osborn R, et al. How does the quality of care compare in five countries? *Health Aff (Millwood).* 2004;23(3):89–99.

15. Midwest Business Group on Health. Reducing the costs of poor-quality health care through responsibly purchasing leadership. 2004. Available at: www.mbgh.org/pdf/ Cost%20of%20Poor%20Quality%20Report.pdf. Accessed December 15, 2004.

16. Gold M, Siegel J, Russell L, Weinstein M. *Cost-Effectiveness in Health and Medicine.* New York: Oxford University Press; 1996.

17. Turnock B. Public Health: *What It Is and How It Works.* Gaithersburg, MD: Aspen; 2001.

18. Saha S, Hoerger T, Pignone M, et al. The art and science of incorporating cost effectiveness into evidence-based recommendations for clinical preventive services. *Am J Prev Med.* 2001;20(3):36–43.

19. Havighurst C. Consumers versus managed care: The new class actions. *Health Aff (Millwood)*. 2004;20(4):8–27.

20. Leapfrog Group, The. Available at: www.leapfroggroup.org. Accessed December 15, 2004.

21. U.S. government. Medicare Prescription Drug, Improvement, and Modernization Act of 2003. Available at: www.cms.hhs.gov/medicareform/. Accessed July 11, 2005.

22. Granados A, Jonsson E, Banta H, et al. EUR-ASSESS project subgroup report on dissemination and impact. *Int J Technol Assess Health Care*. 1997;13(2):220–286.

23. Coulter A. Perspectives on health technology assessment: Response from patient's perspective. *Int J Technol Assess Health Care*. 2004;20(1):92–96.

24. Weatherly H, Drummond M, Smith D. Using evidence in the development of local health policies: Some evidence from the United Kingdom. *Int J Tech Assess Health Care*. 2002;18(4):771–781.

25. Chinitz D. Health technology assessment in four countries: Response from political science. *Int J Technol Assess Health Care*. 2004;20(1):5–60.

26. Smith R. The failings of NICE: time to start work on version 2. *BM J*. 2000;321(7273): 1363–1364.

27. Towse A, Pritchard C. National Institute for Clinical Excellence (NICE): Is economic appraisal working? *Pharmacoeconomics*. 2002;20(3):95–105.

28. Holland W. Health technology assessment and public health: a commentary. *Int J Technol Assess Health Care*. 2004;20(1):77–80.

29. Patented Medicine Prices Review Board. Available at: www.pmprb-cepmb.gc.ca. Accessed December 15, 2004.

30. Menon D. Pharmaceutical cost control in Canada: Does it work? *Health Aff (Millwood)*. 2001;20(3):92–103.

31. Canadian Coordination Office for Health Technology Assessment. Available at: www.ccohta.ca. Accessed December 15, 2004.

32. Pierson R. U.S. seen eventually adopting drug price controls. *Reuters*. 2004.

33. George B, Harris A, Mitchell A. Cost-effectiveness analysis and the consistency of decision making: evidence from pharmaceutical reimbursement in Australia (1991–1996). *Pharmacoeconomics*. 2001;19(11):1103–1109.

34. Hill S, Mitchell A, Henry D. Problems with the interpretation of pharmacoeconomic analyses: A review of submissions to the Australian pharmaceutical benefits scheme. *JAMA*. 2000;283(16):2116–2121.

35. Birkett D, Mitchell A, McManus P. A cost-effectiveness approach to drug subsidy and pricing in Australia. *Health Aff*. 2001;20(3):104–114.

36. Weekes L, Brooks C. Drug and Therapeutics Committees in Australia: Expected and actual performance. *Br J Clin Pharmacol*. 1996;42(5):551–557.

37. Leach D. Competence is a habit. *JAMA*. 2002;287(2):243–244.

38. Accreditation Council for Graduate Medical Education. Available at: www.acgme.org. Accessed December 15, 2004.

INDEX